Comprehensive Keto Air Fryer Diet Cookbook

Fit and Healthy Recipes for Busy People

Rudy Kent

Introduction

What's the difference between an air fryer and deep fryer? Air fryers bake food at a high temperature with a high-powered fan, while deep fryers cook food in a vat of oil that has been heated up to a specific temperature. Both cook food quickly, but an air fryer requires practically zero preheat time while a deep fryer can take upwards of 10 minutes. Air fryers also require little to no oil and deep fryers require a lot that absorb into the food. Food comes out crispy and juicy in both appliances, but don't taste the same, usually because deep fried foods are coated in batter that cook differently in an air fryer vs a deep fryer. Battered foods needs to be sprayed with oil before cooking in an air fryer to help them color and get crispy, while the hot oil soaks into the batter in a deep fryer. Flour-based batters and wet batters don't cook well in an air fryer, but they come out very well in a deep fryer.

The ketogenic diet is one such example. The diet calls for a very small number of carbs to be eaten. This means food such as rice, pasta, and other starchy vegetables like potatoes are off the menu. Even relaxed versions of the keto diet minimize carbs to a large extent and this compromises the goals of many dieters. They end up having to exert large amounts of willpower to follow the diet. This doesn't do them any favors since willpower is like a muscle. At some point, it tires and this is when the dieter goes right back to their old pattern of eating. I have personal experience with this. In terms of health benefits, the keto diet offers the most. The reduction of carbs forces your body to mobilize fat and this results in automatic fat loss and better health.

Feel free to mix and match the recipes you see in here and play around with them. Eating is supposed to be fun! Unfortunately, we've associated fun eating with unhealthy food. This doesn't have to be the case. The air fryer, combined with the Mediterranean diet, will make your mealtimes fun-filled again and full of taste. There's no grease and messy cleanups to deal with anymore. Are you excited yet?

You should be! You're about to embark on a journey full of air fried goodness!

Table of Contents

Famous Blooming Onion with Mayo Dip

Cooking Time:

25 minutes

Serve:3

Ingredients:

1 large Vidalia onion

½ cup all-purpose flour

1 teaspoon salt

½ teaspoon ground black pepper

1 teaspoon cayenne pepper

½ teaspoon dried thyme

½ teaspoon dried oregano

½ teaspoon ground cumin

2 eggs

¼ cup milk

Mayo Dip:

3 tablespoons mayonnaise

3 tablespoons sour cream

1 tablespoon horseradish, drained

Kosher salt and freshly ground black pepper, to taste

Directions:

1.Cut off the top ½ inch of the Vidalia onion; peel your onion and place it cut-side down. Starting ½ inch from the root, cut the onion in half.

2.Make a second cut that splits each half in two. You will have 4 quarters held together by the root.

3.Repeat these cuts, splitting the 4 quarters to yield eighths; then, you should split them again until you have 16 evenly spaced cuts.

4.Turn the onion over and gently separate the outer pieces using your fingers. In a mixing bowl, thoroughly combine the flour and spices.

5.In a separate bowl, whisk the eggs and milk. Dip the onion into the egg mixture, followed by the flour mixture.

6.Spritz the onion with cooking spray and transfer to the lightly greased cooking basket. Cook for 370 degrees F for 12 to 15 minutes. Meanwhile, make the mayo dip by whisking the remaining ingredients. Serve and enjoy!

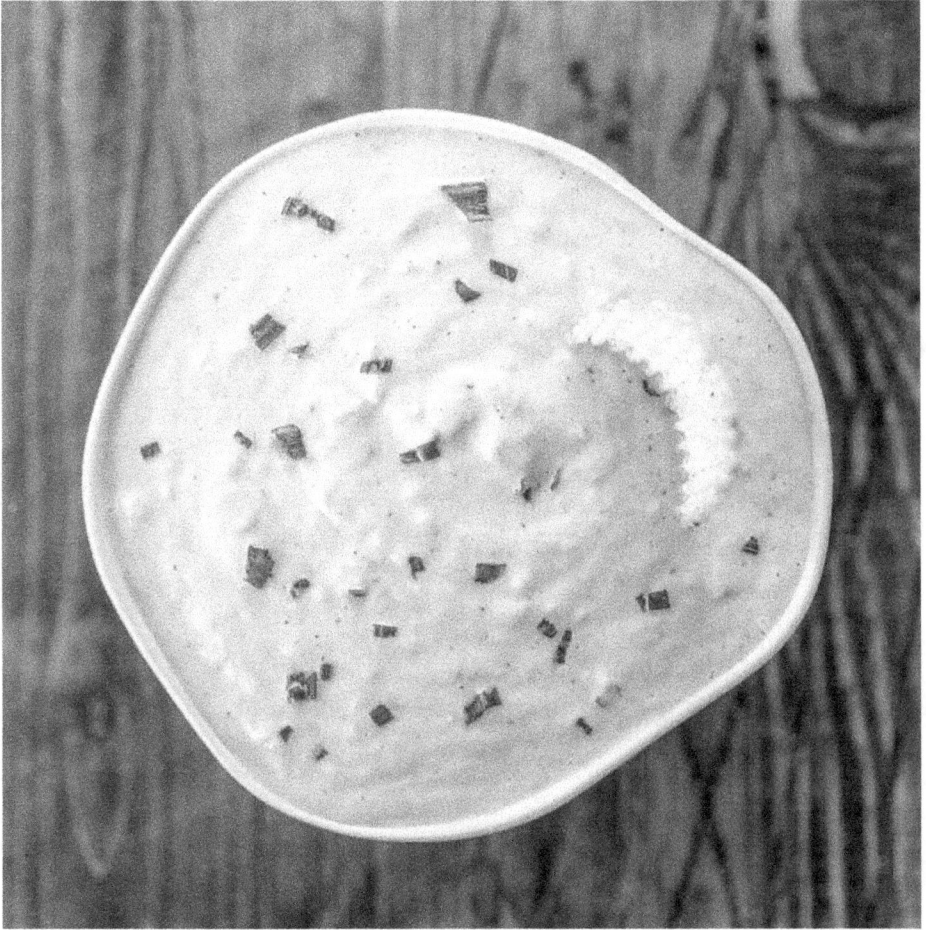

Roasted Parsnip Sticks with Salted Caramel

Cooking Time:

25 minutes

Serve:4

Ingredients:

1 pound parsnip, trimmed, scrubbed, cut into sticks

2 tablespoon avocado oil

2 tablespoons granulated sugar

2 tablespoons butter

¼ teaspoon ground allspice

½ teaspoon coarse salt

Directions:

1.Toss the parsnip with the avocado oil; bake in the preheated Air Fryer at 380 degrees F for 15 minutes, shaking the cooking basket occasionally to ensure even cooking.

2.Then, heat the sugar and 1 tablespoon of water in a small pan over medium heat. Cook until the sugar has dissolved; bring to a boil.

3.Keep swirling the pan around until the sugar reaches a rich caramel color. Pour in 2 tablespoons of cold water. Now, add the butter, allspice, and salt.

4.The mixture should be runny. Afterwards, drizzle the salted caramel over the roasted parsnip sticks and enjoy!

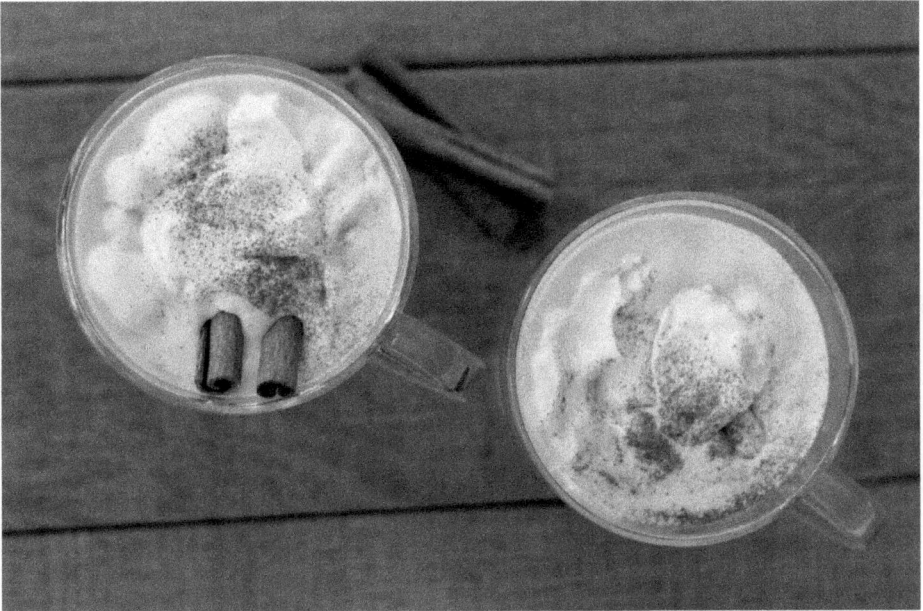

Sea Scallops and Bacon Skewers

Cooking Time:

50 minutes

Serve:6

Ingredients:

½ pound sea scallops

½ cup coconut milk

6 ounces orange juice

1 tablespoon vermouth

Sea salt and ground black pepper, to taste

½ pound bacon, diced

1 shallot, diced

1 teaspoon garlic powder

1 teaspoon paprika

Directions:

1.In a ceramic bowl, place the sea scallops, coconut milk, orange juice, vermouth, salt, and black pepper; let it marinate for 30 minutes.

2.Assemble the skewers alternating the scallops, bacon, and shallots. Sprinkle garlic powder and paprika all over the skewers.

3.Bake in the preheated air Fryer at 400 degrees F for 6 minutes. Serve warm and enjoy!

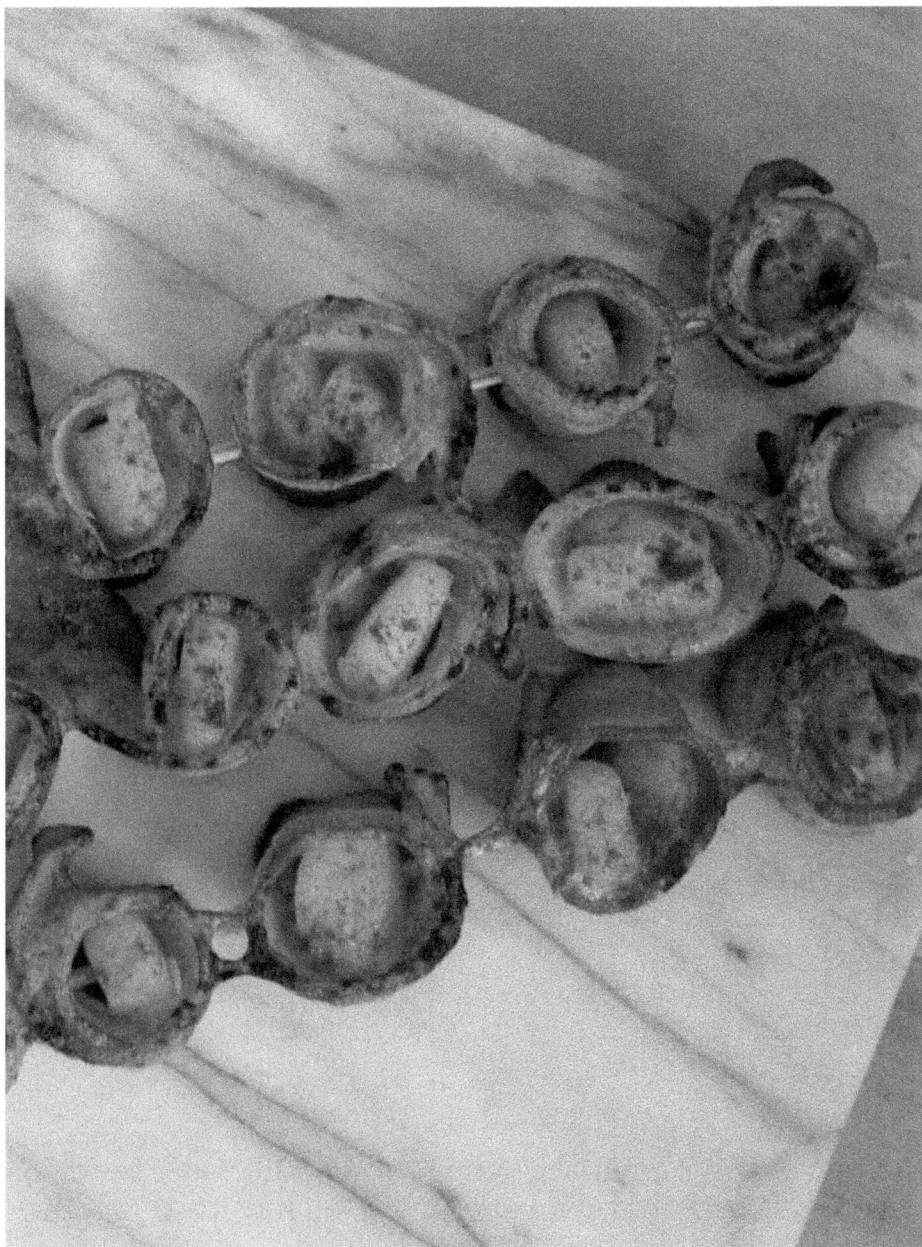

Summer Meatball Skewers

Cooking Time:

20 minutes

Serve:4

Ingredients:
½ pound ground pork
½ pound ground beef
1 teaspoon dried onion flakes
1 teaspoon fresh garlic, minced
1 teaspoon dried parsley flakes
Salt and black pepper, to taste
1 red pepper, 1-inch pieces
1 cup pearl onions
½ cup barbecue sauce

Directions:

1.Mix the ground meat with the onion flakes, garlic, parsley flakes, salt, and black pepper. Shape the mixture into 1- inch balls.

2.Thread the meatballs, pearl onions, and peppers alternately onto skewers. Microwave the barbecue sauce for 10 seconds.

3.Cook in the preheated Air Fryer at 380 degrees for 5 minutes. Turn the skewers over halfway through the cooking time.

4.Brush with the sauce and cook for a further 5 minutes. Work in batches. Serve with the remaining barbecue sauce and enjoy!

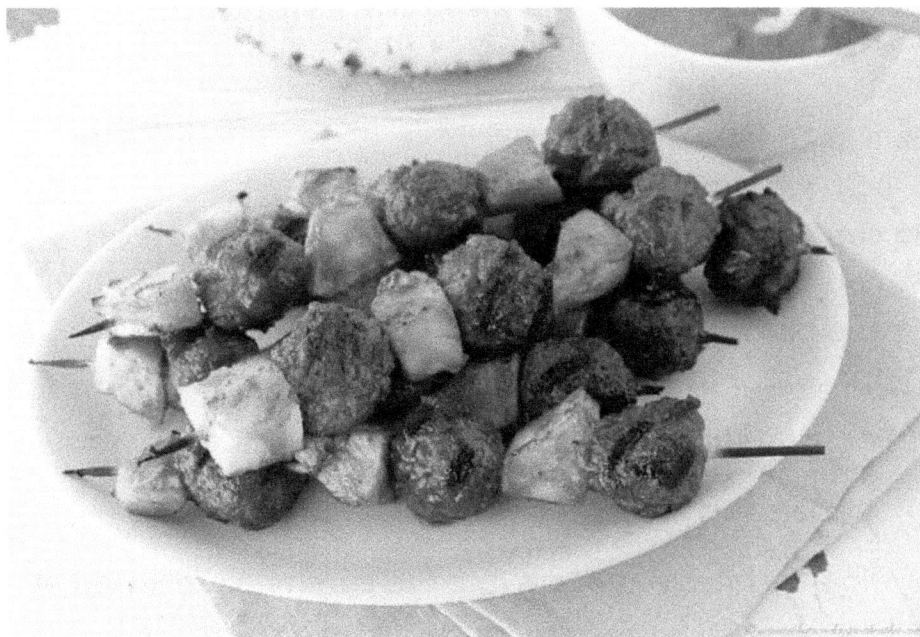

Chicken Nuggets with Campfire Sauce

Cooking Time:

20 minutes

Serve:6

Ingredients:

1 pound chicken breasts, slice into tenders
½ teaspoon cayenne pepper
Salt and black pepper, to taste
¼ cup cornmeal
1 egg, whisked
½ cup seasoned breadcrumbs
¼ cup mayo
¼ cup barbecue sauce

Directions:

1.Pat the chicken tenders dry with a kitchen towel. Season with the cayenne pepper, salt, and black pepper.

2.Dip the chicken tenders into the cornmeal, followed by the egg. Press the chicken tenders into the breadcrumbs, coating evenly.

3.Place the chicken tenders in the lightly greased Air Fryer basket. Cook at 360 degrees for 9 to 12 minutes, turning them over to cook evenly.

4.In a mixing bowl, thoroughly combine the mayonnaise with the barbecue sauce. Serve the chicken nuggets with the sauce for dipping. Enjoy!

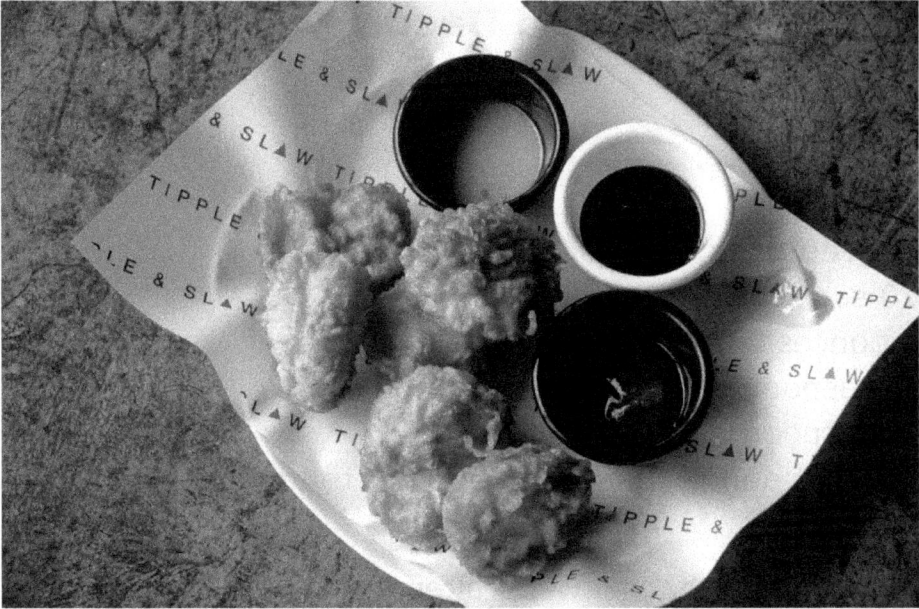

Sea Scallops and Bacon Kabobs

Cooking Time:

10 minutes

Serve:4

Ingredients:

10 sea scallops, frozen

4 ounces bacon, diced

1 teaspoon garlic powder

1 teaspoon paprika

Sea salt and ground black pepper, to taste

Directions:

1.Assemble the skewers alternating sea scallops and bacon. Sprinkle the garlic powder, paprika, salt and black pepper all over your kabobs.

2.Bake your kabobs in the preheated Air Fryer at 400 degrees F for 6 minutes. Serve warm with your favorite sauce for dipping. Enjoy!

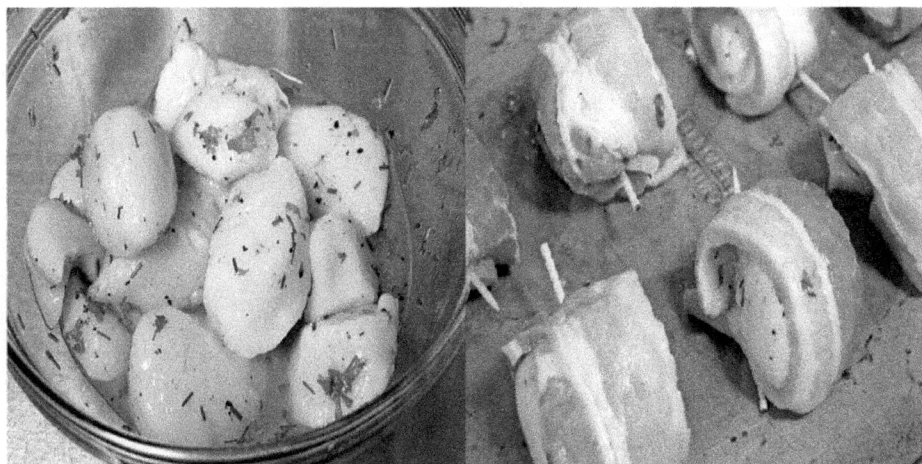

Chili-Lime French Fries

Cooking Time:

20 minutes

Serve:4

Ingredients:

1pound potatoes, peeled and cut into matchsticks

1 teaspoon olive oil

1 lime, freshly squeezed

1 teaspoon chili powder

Sea salt and ground black pepper, to taste

Directions:

1.Toss your potatoes with the remaining ingredients until well coated.

2.Transfer your potatoes to the Air Fryer cooking basket. Cook the French fries at 370 degrees F for 9 minutes.

3.Shake the cooking basket and continue to cook for about 9 minutes. Serve immediately. Enjoy!

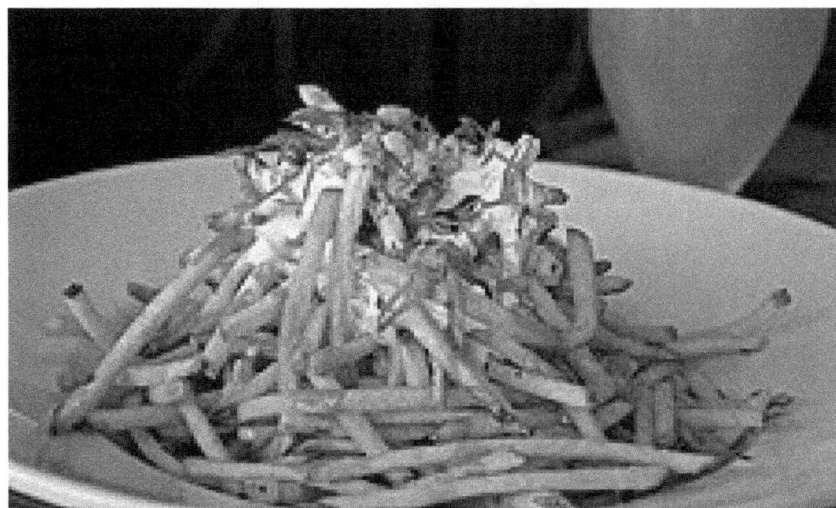

Easy Toasted Nuts

Cooking Time:
10 minutes
Serve:3
Ingredients:
½ cup pecans
1 cup almonds
2 tablespoons egg white
1 tablespoon granulated sugar
A pinch of coarse sea salt

Directions:

1.Toss the pecans and almonds with the egg white, granulated sugar and salt until well coated.

2.Transfer the pecans and almonds to the Air Fryer cooking basket.

3.Roast the pecans and almonds at 360 degrees F for about 6 to 7 minutes, shaking the basket once or twice. Taste and adjust seasonings. Enjoy!

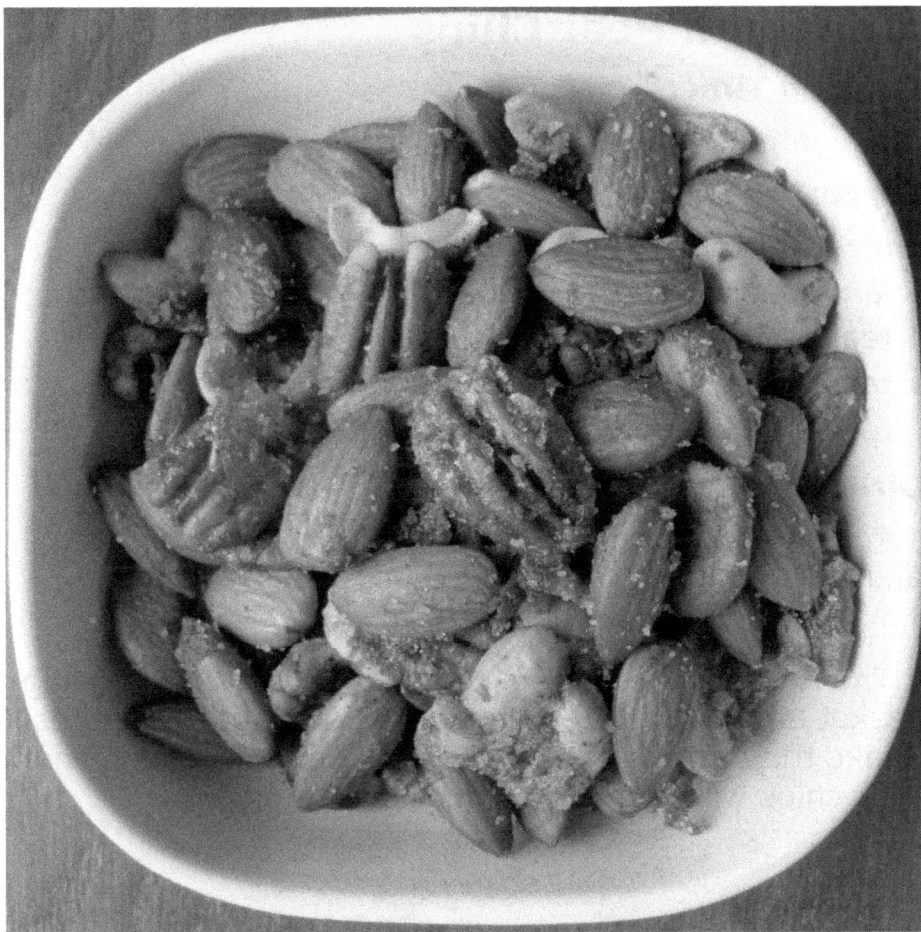

Cinnamon Pear Chips

Cooking Time:

10 minutes

Serve:2

Ingredients:

1 large pear, cored and sliced

1 teaspoon apple pie spice blend

1 teaspoon coconut oil

1 teaspoon honey

Directions:

1.Toss the pear slices with the spice blend, coconut oil and honey.

2.Then, place the pear slices in the Air Fryer cooking basket and cook at 360 degrees F for about 8 minutes. Shake the basket once or twice to ensure even cooking. Pear chips will crisp up as it cools. Enjoy!

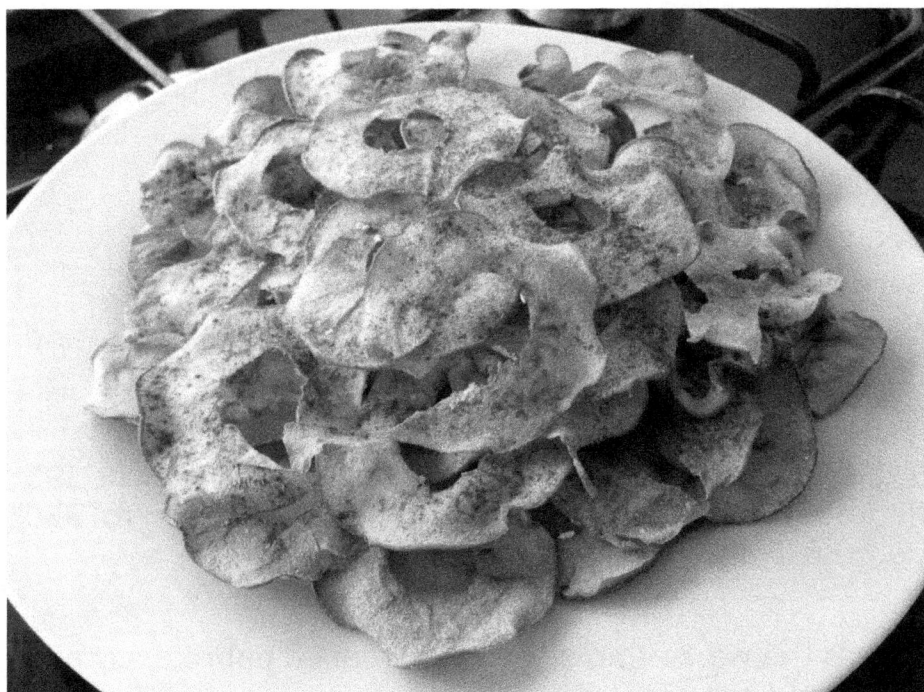

Crunchy Roasted Chickpeas

Cooking Time:

20 minutes

Serve: 3

Ingredients:

1 tablespoon extra-virgin olive oil

8 ounces can chickpeas, drained

½ teaspoon smoked paprika

½ teaspoon ground cumin

½ teaspoon garlic powder

Sea salt, to taste

Directions:

1.Drizzle olive oil over the drained chickpeas and transfer them to the Air Fryer cooking basket.

2. Cook your chickpeas in the preheated Air Fryer at 395 degrees F for 13 minutes. Turn your Air Fryer to 350 degrees F and cook an additional 6 minutes.

3.Toss the warm chickpeas with smoked paprika, cumin, garlic and salt. Enjoy!

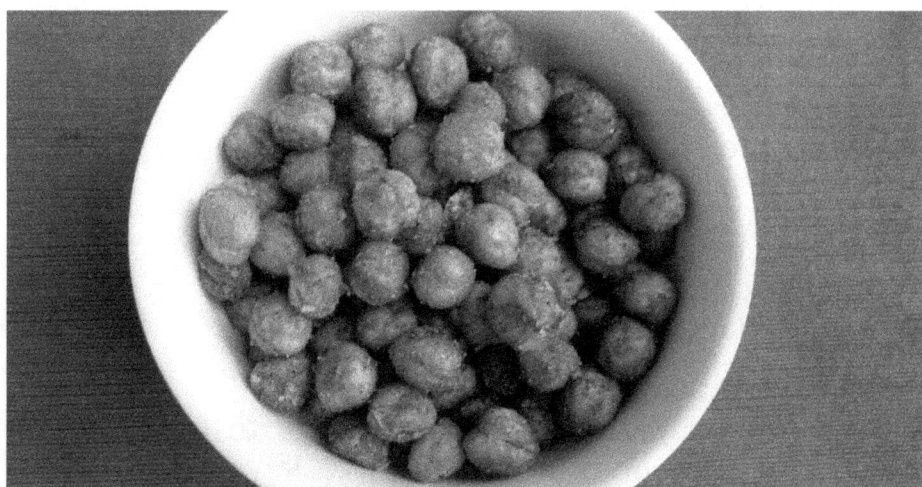

Baked Cheese Crisps

Cooking Time:

15 minutes

Serve:4

Ingredients:

½ cup Parmesan cheese, shredded

1 cup Cheddar cheese, shredded

1 teaspoon Italian seasoning

½ cup marinara sauce

Directions:

1.Start by preheating your Air Fryer to 350 degrees F. Place a piece of parchment paper in the cooking basket.

2.Mix the cheese with the Italian seasoning. Add about 1 tablespoon of the cheese mixture per crisp to the basket, making sure they are not touching.

3.Bake for 6 minutes or until browned to your liking. Work in batches and place them on a large tray to cool slightly. Serve with the marinara sauce. Enjoy!

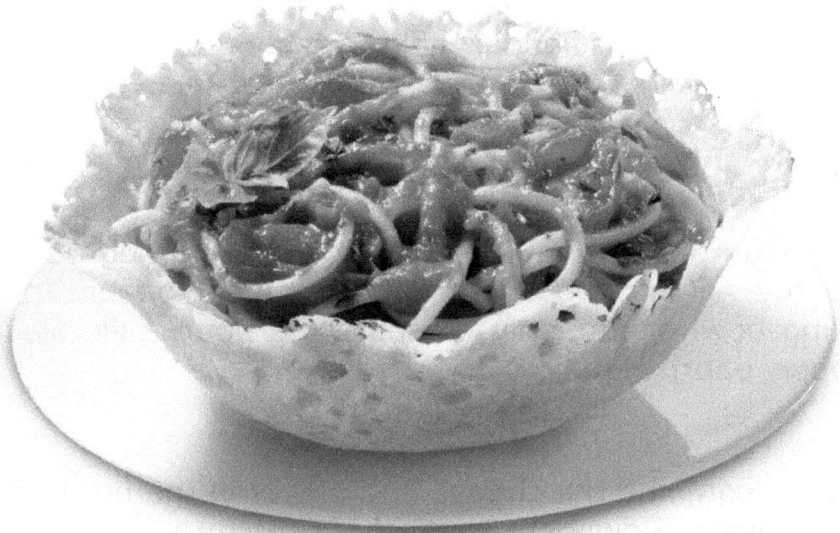

Southern Cheese Straws

Cooking Time:

30 minutes

Serve:6

Ingredients:

1 cup all-purpose flour

Sea salt and ground black pepper, to taste

¼ teaspoon smoked paprika

½ teaspoon celery seeds

4 ounces mature Cheddar, cold, freshly grated

1 sticks butter

Directions:

1.Start by preheating your air Fryer to 330 degrees F. Line the Air Fryer basket with parchment paper. In a mixing bowl, thoroughly combine the flour, salt, black pepper, paprika, and celery seeds.

2.Then, combine the cheese and butter in the bowl of a stand mixer. Slowly stir in the flour mixture and mix to combine well.

3.Then, pack the dough into a cookie press fitted with a star disk. Pipe the long ribbons of dough across the parchment paper.

4.Then cut into six-inch lengths. Bake in the preheated Air Fryer for 15 minutes. Repeat with the remaining dough. Let the cheese straws cool on a rack. You can store them between sheets of parchment in an airtight container. Enjoy!

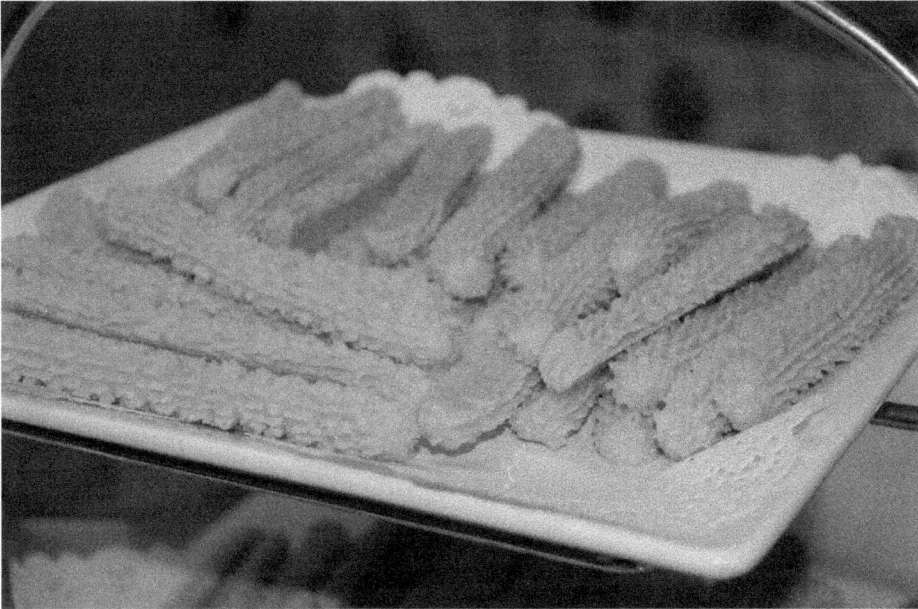

Crunchy Broccoli Fries

Cooking Time:

15 minutes

Serve:4

Ingredients:

1 pound broccoli florets
½ teaspoon onion powder
1 teaspoon granulated garlic
½ teaspoon cayenne pepper
Sea salt and ground black pepper, to taste
2 tablespoons sesame oil
4 tablespoons parmesan cheese, preferably freshly grated

Directions:

1.Start by preheating the Air Fryer to 400 degrees F. Blanch the broccoli in salted boiling water until al dente, about 3 to 4 minutes.

2.Drain well and transfer to the lightly greased Air Fryer basket. Add the onion powder, garlic, cayenne pepper, salt, black pepper, and sesame oil.

3.Cook for 6 minutes, tossing halfway through the cooking time. Serve and enjoy!

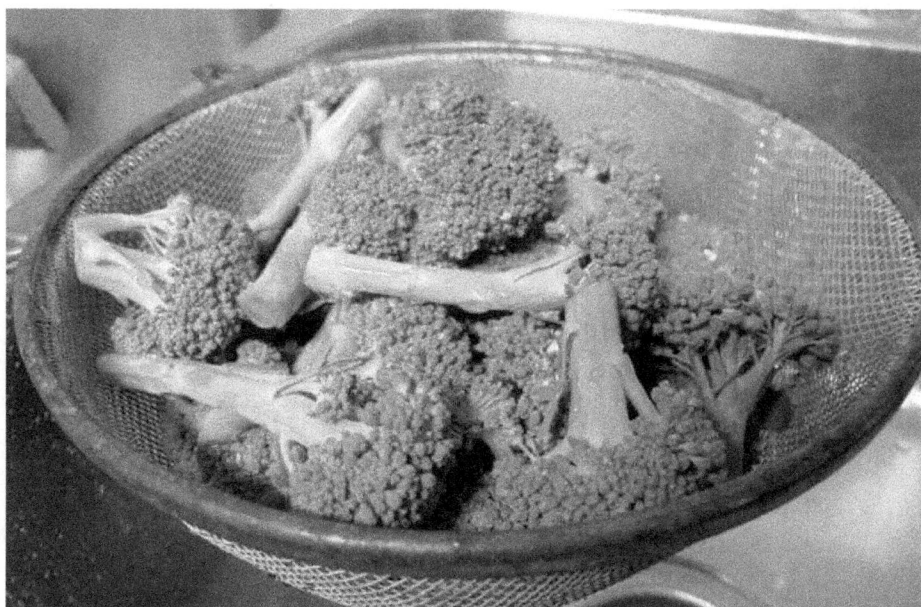

Beer Battered Vidalia Rings

Cooking Time:

30 minutes

Serve:4

Ingredients:

½ pound Vidalia onions, sliced into rings

½ cup all-purpose flour

¼ cup cornmeal

½ teaspoon baking powder

Sea salt and freshly cracked black pepper, to taste

¼ teaspoon garlic powder

2 eggs, beaten

½ cup lager-style beer

1 cup plain breadcrumbs

2 tablespoons peanut oil

Directions:

1.Place the onion rings in the bowl with icy cold water; let them soak approximately 20 minutes; drain the onion rings and pat them dry.

2.In a shallow bowl, mix the flour, cornmeal, baking powder, salt, and black pepper.

3.Add the garlic powder, eggs and beer; mix well to combine. In another shallow bowl, mix the breadcrumbs with the peanut oil.

4.Dip the onion rings in the flour/egg mixture; then, dredge in the breadcrumb mixture. Roll to coat them evenly. Spritz the Air Fryer basket with cooking spray;

arrange the breaded onion rings in the basket. Cook in the preheated Air Fryer at 400 degrees F for 4 to 5 minutes, turning them over halfway through the cooking time. Enjoy!

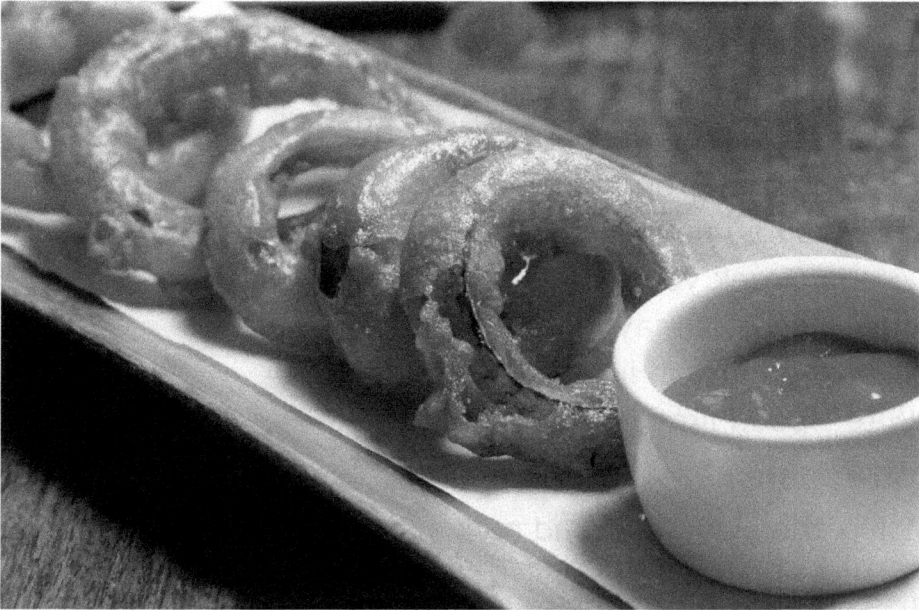

Avocado Fries with Lime Sauce

Cooking Time:

15 minutes

Serve:4

Ingredients:

½ cup plain flour
½ milk
½ cup tortilla chips, crushed
½ teaspoon red pepper flakes, crushed
Sea salt and ground black pepper, to taste
2 avocados, peeled, pitted and sliced
½ cup Greek yogurt
4 tablespoons mayonnaise
1 teaspoon fresh lime juice
½ teaspoon lime chili seasoning salt

Directions:

1.Mix the plain flour and milk in a plate. Add the crushed tortilla chips, red pepper flakes, salt and black pepper to another rimmed plate.

2.Dredge the avocado slices in the flour mixture and then, coat them in the crushed tortilla chips. Cook the avocado at 390 degrees F for about 8 minutes, shaking the basket halfway through the cooking time.

3.In the meantime, mix the remaining ingredients, until well combined. Serve warm avocado fries with the lime sauce. Enjoy!

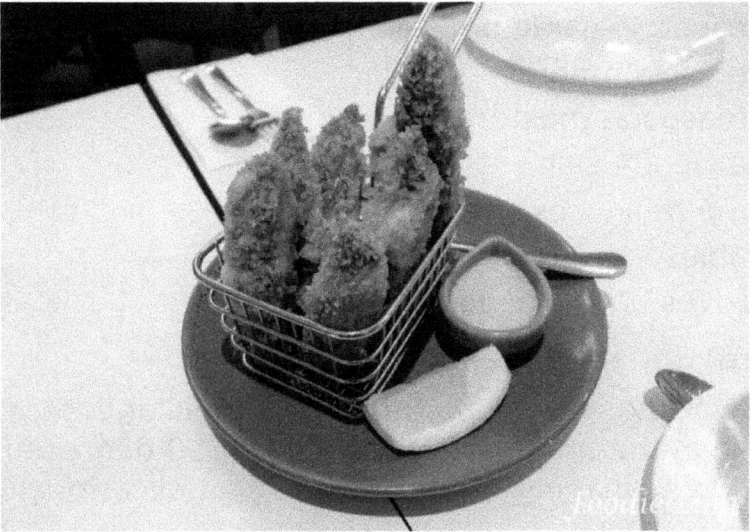

Kale Chips with Tahini Sauce

Cooking Time:

15 minutes

Serve:4

Ingredients

5 cups kale leaves, torn into
1-inch pieces
1 ½ tablespoons sesame oil
½ teaspoon shallot powder
1 teaspoon garlic powder
¼ teaspoon porcini powder
½ teaspoon mustard seeds
1 teaspoon salt
⅓ cup tahini sesame butter
1 tablespoon fresh lemon juice
2 cloves garlic, minced

Directions:

1.Toss the kale with the sesame oil and seasonings. Bake in the preheated Air Fryer at 350 degrees F for 10 minutes, shaking the cooking basket occasionally.

2.Bake until the edges are brown. Work in batches. Meanwhile, make the sauce by whisking all ingredients in a small mixing bowl. Serve and enjoy!

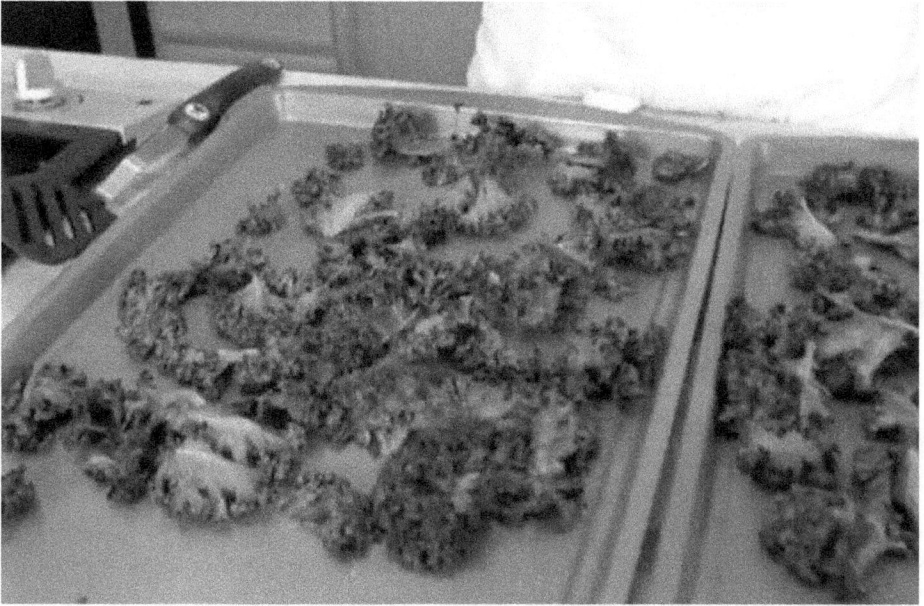

Thyme-Roasted Sweet Potatoes

Cooking Time:

35 minutes

Serve:3

Ingredients:

1pound sweet potatoes, peeled, cut into bite-sized pieces

2 tablespoons olive oil

1 teaspoon sea salt

¼ teaspoon freshly ground black pepper

½ teaspoon cayenne pepper

2 fresh thyme sprigs

Directions:

1.Arrange the potato slices in a single layer in the lightly greased cooking basket.

2.Add the olive oil, salt, black pepper, and cayenne pepper; toss to coat.

3.Bake at 380 degrees F for 30 minutes, shaking the cooking basket occasionally. Bake until tender and slightly browned, working in batches. Serve warm, garnished with thyme sprigs.

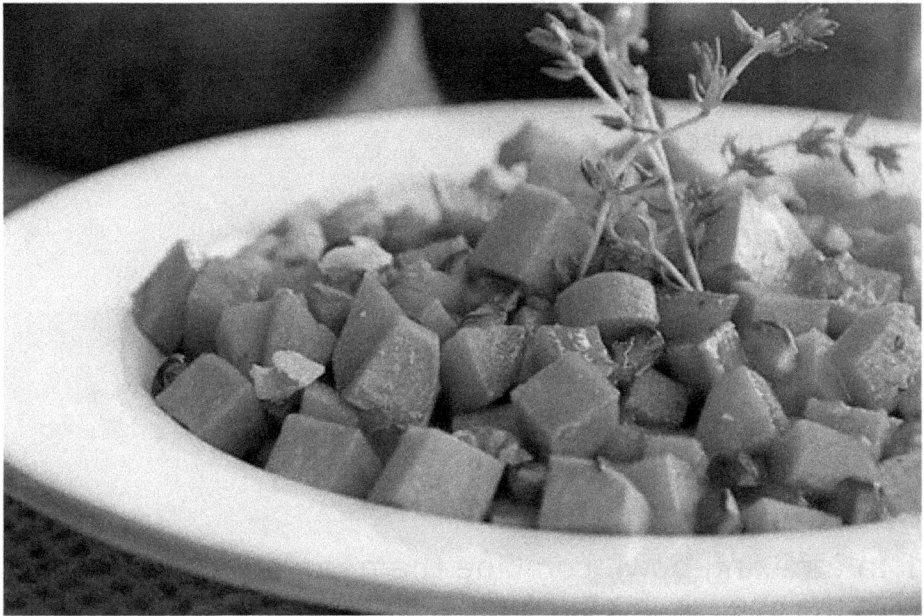

Cocktail Cranberry Meatballs

Cooking Time:

35 minutes

Serve:6

Ingredients:

½ pound ground beef

½ pound ground turkey

¼ cup Parmesan cheese, grated

¼ cup breadcrumbs

1 small shallot, chopped

2 eggs, whisked

½ teaspoon garlic powder

½ teaspoon porcini powder

Sea salt and ground black pepper, to taste

1 teaspoon red pepper flakes, crushed

1 tablespoon soy sauce

1 8-ounce can jellied cranberry sauce

6 ounces tomato-based chili sauce

Directionbs:

1.In a mixing bowl, combine the ground meat together with the cheese, breadcrumbs, shallot, eggs, and spices. Shape the mixture into 1-inch balls.

2.Cook the meatballs in the preheated Air Fryer at 380 degrees for 5 minutes.

3.Shake halfway through the cooking time. Work in batches.

4.Whisk the soy sauce, cranberry sauce, and chili sauce in a mixing bowl. Pour the sauce over the meatballs and bake an additional 2 minutes. Serve with cocktail sticks. Enjoy!

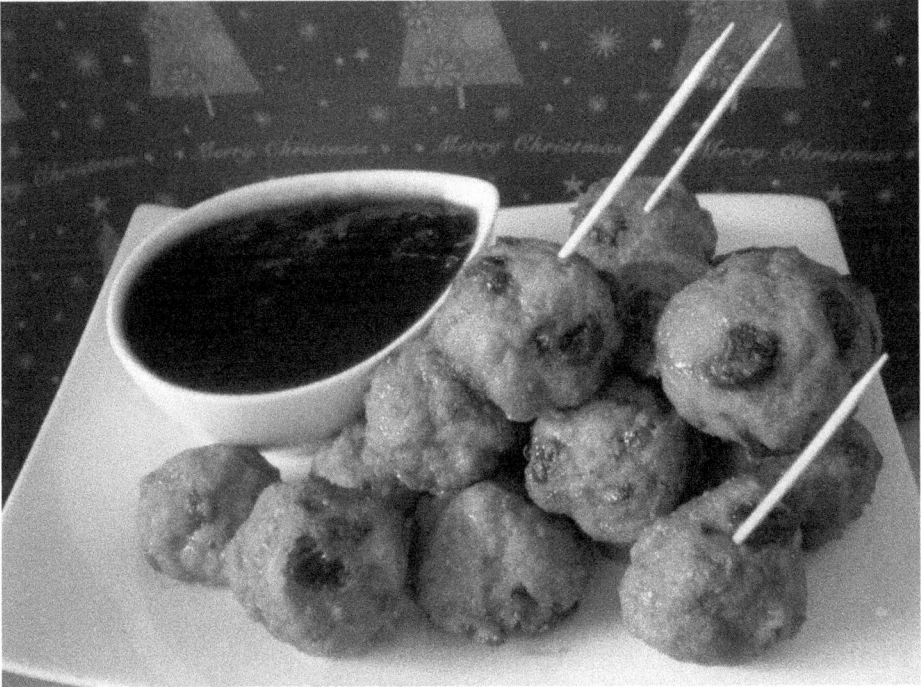

Teriyaki Chicken Drumettes

Cooking Time:

25 minutes

Serve: 3

Ingredients:

1½ pounds chicken drumettes

Sea salt and cracked black pepper, to taste

2 tablespoons fresh chives, roughly chopped Teriyaki Sauce:

1 tablespoon sesame oil

¼ cup soy sauce

½ cup water

¼ cup honey

½ teaspoon Five-spice powder

2 tablespoons rice wine vinegar

½ teaspoon fresh ginger, grated

2 cloves garlic, crushed

1 tablespoon corn starch dissolved in

3 tablespoons of water

Directions:

1.Start by preheating your Air Fryer to 380 degrees F. Rub the chicken drumettes with salt and cracked black pepper.

2.Cook in the preheated Air Fryer approximately 15 minutes. Turn them over and cook an additional 7 minutes.

3.While the chicken drumettes are roasting, combine the sesame oil, soy sauce, water, honey, Five-spice powder, vinegar, ginger, and garlic in a pan over medium heat.

4.Cook for 5 minutes, stirring occasionally. Add the cornstarch slurry, reduce the heat, and let it simmer until the glaze thickens.

5.After that, brush the glaze all over the chicken drumettes. Air-fry for a further 6 minutes or until the surface is crispy. Serve topped with the remaining glaze and garnished with fresh chives. Enjoy!

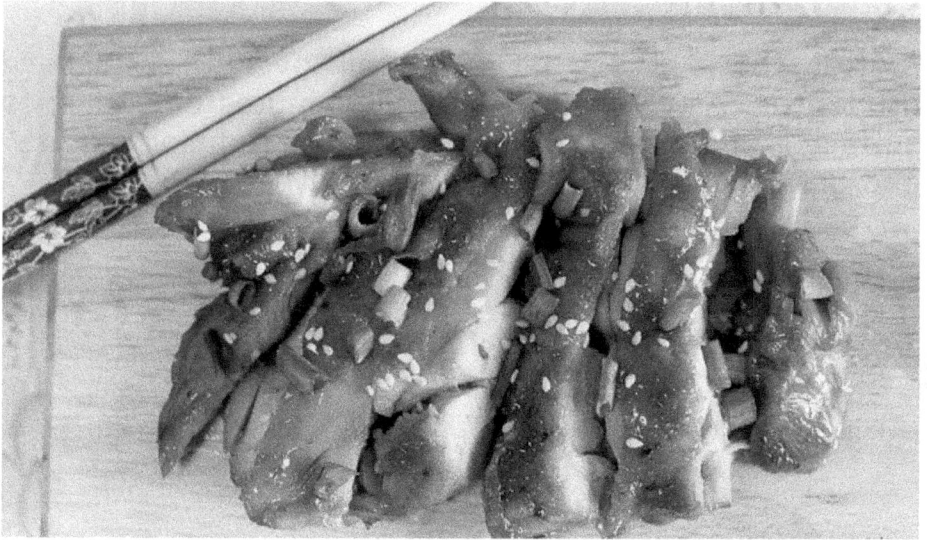

Blue Cheesy Potato Wedges

Cooking Time:

20 minutes

Serve:4

Ingredients:

1Yukon Gold potatoes, peeled and cut into wedges
2 tablespoons ranch seasoning Kosher salt, to taste
½ cup blue cheese, crumbled

Directions:

1.Sprinkle the potato wedges with the ranch seasoning and salt. Grease generously the Air Fryer basket.

2.Place the potatoes in the cooking basket. Roast in the preheated Air Fryer at 400 degrees for 12 minutes.

3.Top with the cheese and roast an additional 3 minutes or until cheese begins to melt. Serve and enjoy!

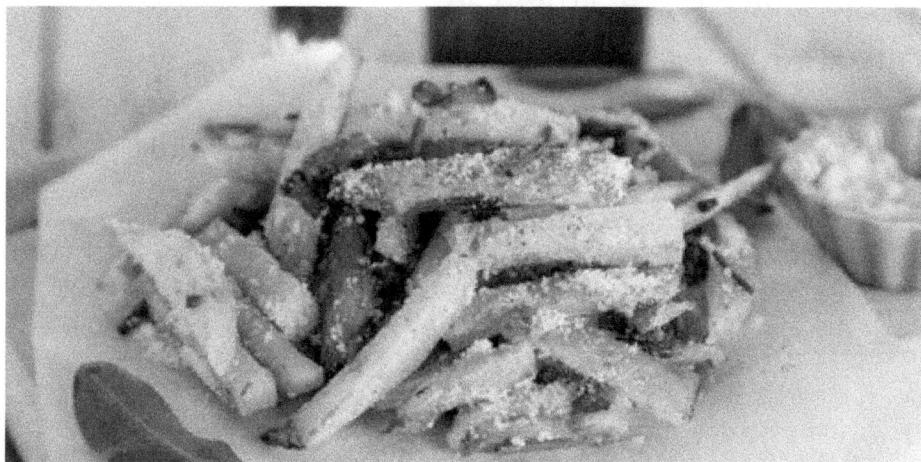

Yakitori Japanese Chicken Skewers

Cooking Time:

30 minutes

Serve:4

Ingredients:

½ pound chicken tenders, cut bite-sized pieces

1 clove garlic, minced

1 teaspoon coriander seeds

Sea salt and ground pepper, to taste

2 tablespoons Shoyu sauce

2 tablespoons sake

1 tablespoon fresh lemon juice

1 teaspoon sesame oil

Directions:

1.Place the chicken tenders, garlic, coriander, salt, black pepper, Shoyu sauce, sake, and lemon juice in a ceramic dish; cover and let it marinate for 2 hours.

2.Then, discard the marinade and tread the chicken tenders onto bamboo skewers. Place the skewered chicken in the lightly greased Air Fryer basket. Drizzle sesame oil all over the skewered chicken.

3.Cook at 360 degrees for 6 minutes. Turn the skewered chicken over; brush with the reserved marinade and cook for a further 6 minutes. Enjoy!

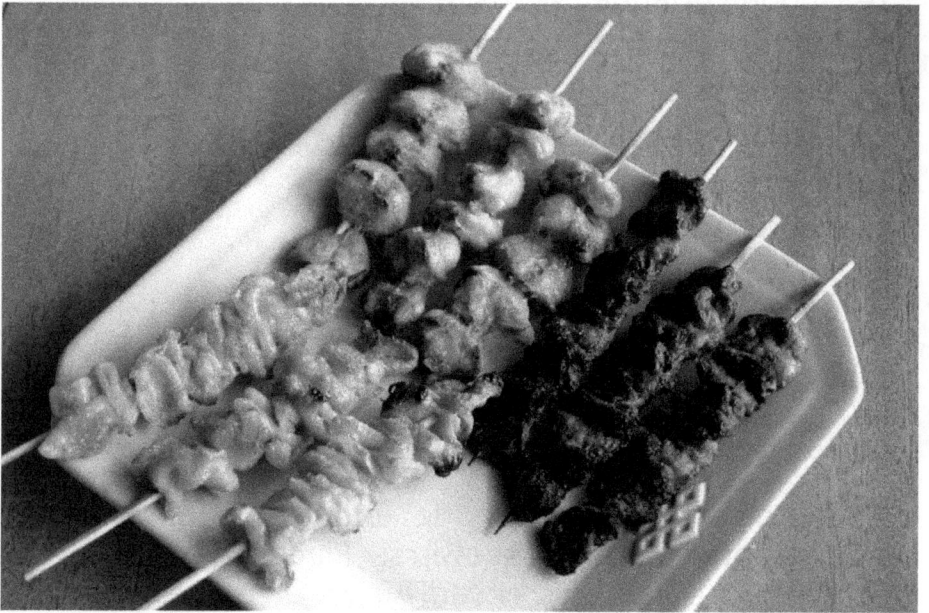

Pecorino Romano Meatballs

Cooking Time:

15 minutes

Serve:2

Ingredients:

½ pound ground turkey

2 tablespoons tomato ketchup

1 teaspoon stone-ground mustard

2 tablespoons scallions, chopped

1 garlic clove, minced

¼ Pecorino-Romano cheese, grated

1 egg, beaten

½ teaspoon red pepper flakes, crushed

Sea salt and ground black pepper, to taste

Directions:

1.In a mixing bowl, thoroughly combine all ingredients. Shape the mixture into 6 equal meatballs.

2.Transfer the meatballs to the Air Fryer cooking basket that is previously greased with a nonstick cooking spray.

3.Cook the meatballs at 360 degrees F for 10 to 11 minutes, shaking the basket occasionally to ensure even cooking.

4.An instant thermometer should read 165 degrees F and serve

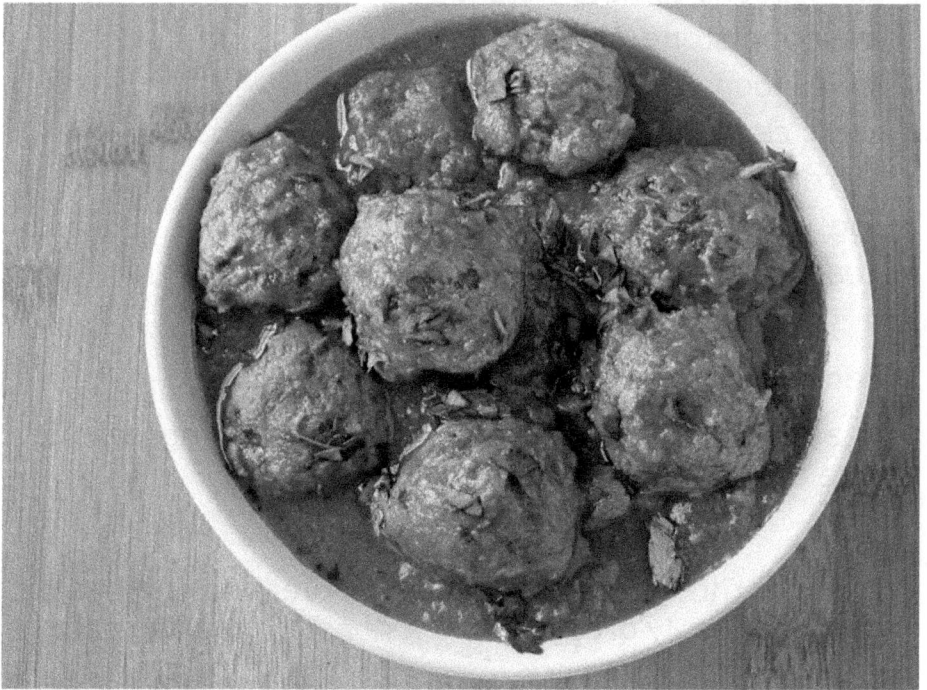

Romano Cheese and Broccoli Balls

Cooking Time:

25 minutes

Serve:4

Ingredients:

½ pound broccoli

½ cup Romano cheese, grated

2 garlic cloves, minced

1 shallot, chopped

4 eggs, beaten

2 tablespoons butter, at room temperature

½ teaspoon paprika

¼ teaspoon dried basil

Sea salt and ground black pepper, to taste

Directions:

Add the broccoli to your food processor and pulse until the consistency resembles rice.

2.Stir in the remaining ingredients; mix until everything is well combined.

3.Shape the mixture into bite-sized balls and transfer them to the lightly greased cooking basket. Cook in the preheated Air Fryer at 375 degrees F for 16 minutes, shaking halfway through the cooking time.

4.Serve with cocktail sticks and tomato ketchup on the side.

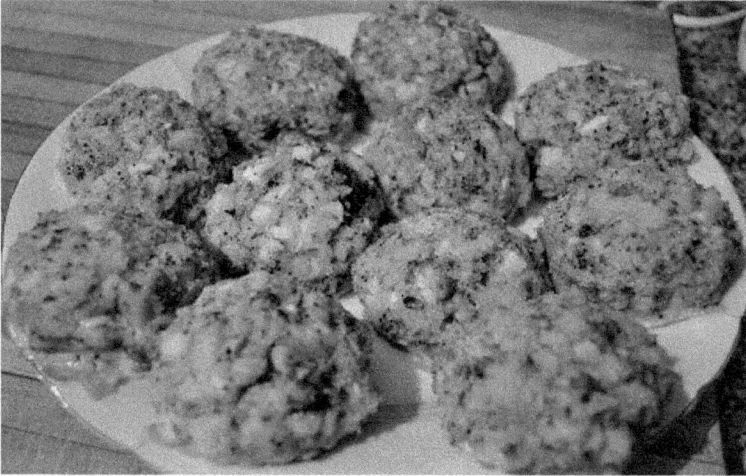

Paprika and Cheese French Fries

Cooking Time:

15 minutes

Serve:4

Ingredients:

8 ounces French fries, frozen

½ cup Monterey-Jack cheese, grated

1 teaspoon paprika Sea salt, to taste

Directions:

1.Cook the French fries in your Air Fryer at 400 degrees F for about 7 minutes.

2.Shake the basket and continue to cook for a further 6 minutes.

3.Top the French fries with cheese, paprika and salt cheese. Continue to cook for 1 minute more or until the cheese has melted. Serve warm and enjoy!

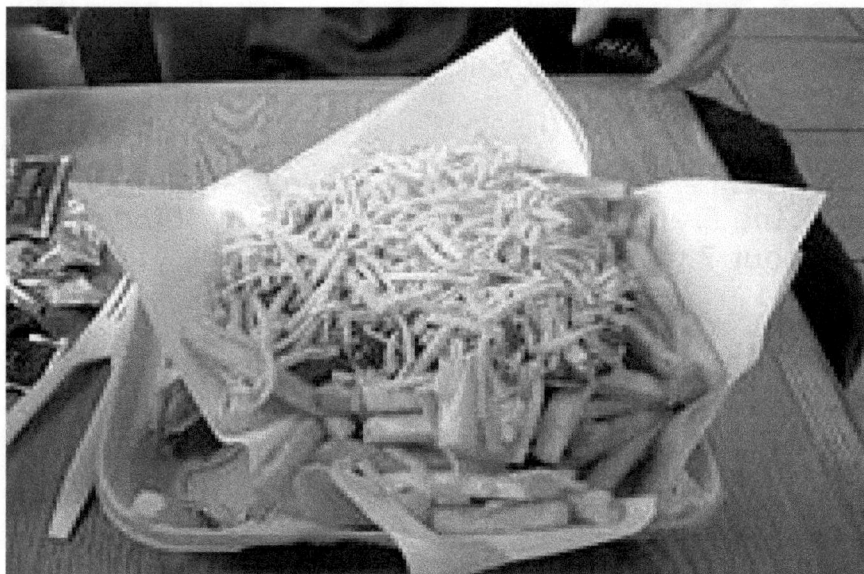

Hot Cheesy Mushrooms Bites

Cooking Time:

20 minutes

Serve:4

Ingredients:

1 teaspoon butter, melted

1 teaspoon fresh garlic, finely minced

4 ounces cheddar cheese, grated

4 tablespoons tortilla chips, crushed

1 tablespoon fresh coriander, chopped

½ teaspoon hot sauce

12 button mushrooms, stalks removed and chopped

Sea salt and ground black pepper, to taste

Directions:

1.In a mixing bowl, thoroughly combine the butter, garlic, cheddar cheese, tortilla chips, coriander, hot sauce and chopped mushrooms.

2.Divide the filling among mushroom caps and transfer them to the air Fryer cooking basket; season them with salt and black pepper.

3.Cook your mushrooms in the preheated Air Fryer at 400 degrees F for 5 minutes. Transfer the warm mushrooms to a serving platter and serve at room temperature. Serve and enjoy!

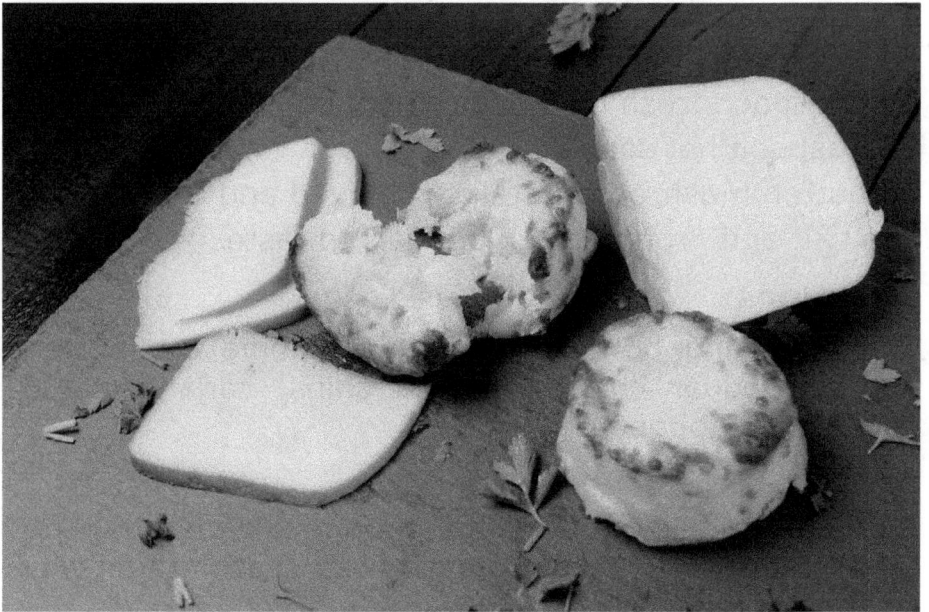

Pork Crackling with Sriracha Dip

Cooking Time:

40 minutes

Serve:3

Ingredients:

½ pound pork rind

Sea salt and ground black pepper, to taste

½ cup tomato sauce

1 teaspoon Sriracha sauce

½ teaspoon stone-ground mustard

Directions:

1.Rub sea salt and pepper on the skin side of the pork rind.

2.Allow it to sit for 30 minutes. Then, cut the pork rind into chunks using kitchen scissors. Roast the pork rind at 380 degrees F for 8 minutes; turn them over and cook for a further 8 minutes or until blistered.

3.Meanwhile, mix the tomato sauce with the Sriracha sauce and mustard. Serve the pork crackling with the Sriracha dip and enjoy

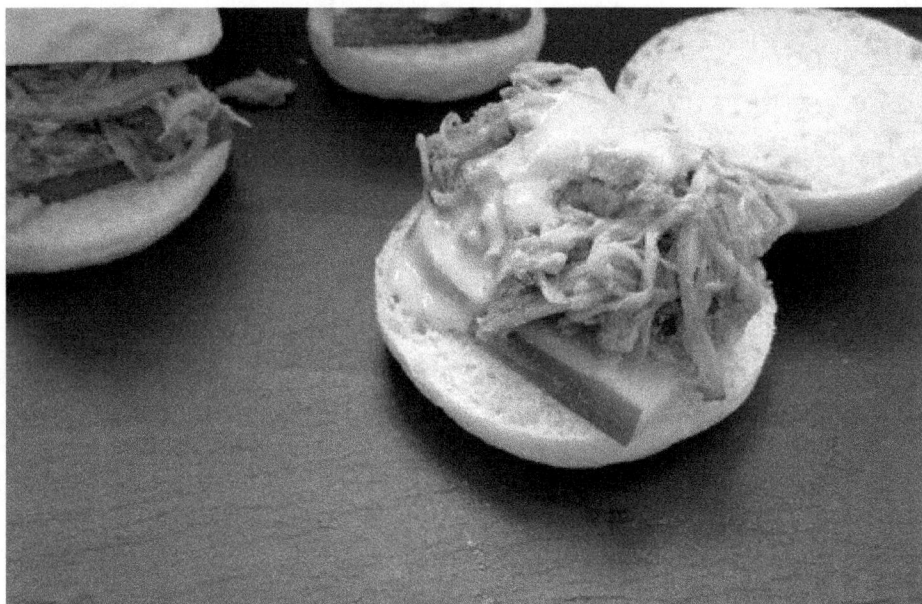

Cheesy Potato Puffs

Cooking Time:

15 minutes

Serve:4

Ingredients:

8 ounces potato puffs

1 teaspoon olive oil4 ounces cheddar cheese, shredded
½ cup tomato sauce

1 teaspoon Dijon mustard

½ teaspoon Italian seasoning mix

Directions:

1.Brush the potato puffs with olive oil and transfer them to the Air Fryer cooking basket. Cook the potato puffs at 400 degrees F for 10 minutes, shaking the basket occasionally to ensure even browning.

2.Top them with cheese and continue to cook for 2 minutes more until the cheese melts. Meanwhile, whisk the tomato sauce with the mustard and Italian seasoning mix.

3.Serve the warm potato puffs with cocktail sticks and the sauce on the side. Serve warm.

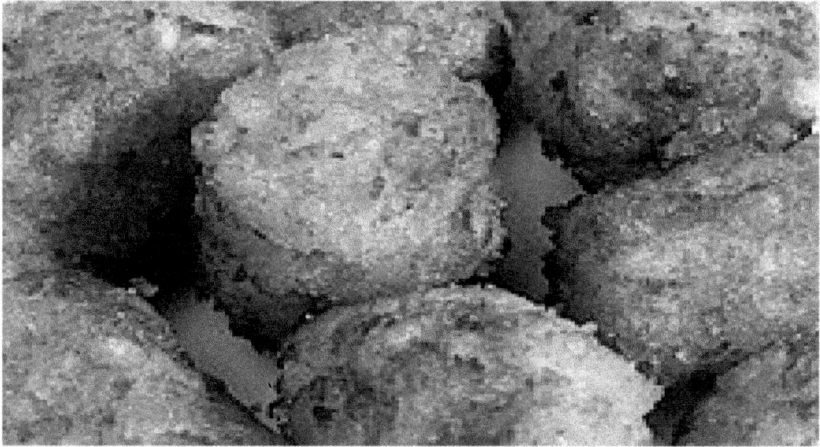

Pepper and Bacon Mini Skewers

Cooking Time:

10 minutes

Serve:4

Ingredients:

4 ounces bacon, diced

2 bell peppers, sliced

¼ cup barbecue sauce

1 teaspoon Ranch seasoning blend

½ cup tomato sauce

1 teaspoon jalapeno, minced

Directions:

1.Assemble the skewers alternating bacon and bell pepper.

2.Toss them with barbecue sauce and Ranch seasoning blend.

3.Cook the mini skewers in the preheated Air Fryer at 400 degrees F for 6 minutes. Mix the tomato sauce and minced jalapeno. Bon appétit!

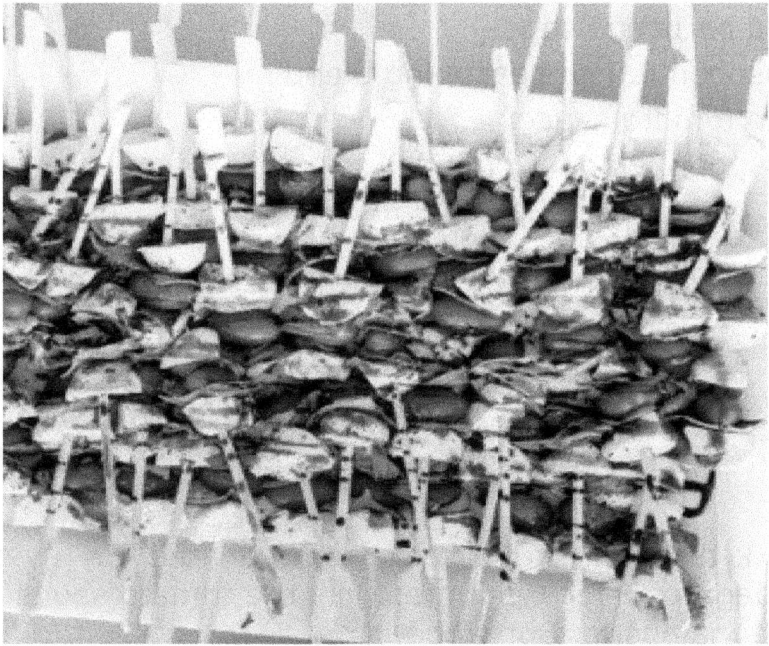

Wonton Sausage Appetizers

Cooking Time:

10 minutes

Serve:5

Ingredients:

½ pound ground sausage

2 tablespoons scallions, chopped

1 garlic clove, minced

½ tablespoon fish sauce

1 teaspoon Sriracha sauce

20 wonton wrappers

1 egg, whisked with

1 tablespoon water

Directions:

1.In a mixing bowl, thoroughly combine the ground sausage, scallions, garlic, fish sauce, and Sriracha.

2.Divide the mixture between the wonton wrappers. Dip your fingers in the egg wash Fold the wonton in half. Bring up the 2 ends of the wonton and use the egg wash to stick them together.

3.Pinch the edges and coat each wonton with the egg wash. Place the folded wontons in the lightly greased cooking basket.

4.Cook at 360 degrees F for 10 minutes. Work in batches and serve warm. Serve warm.

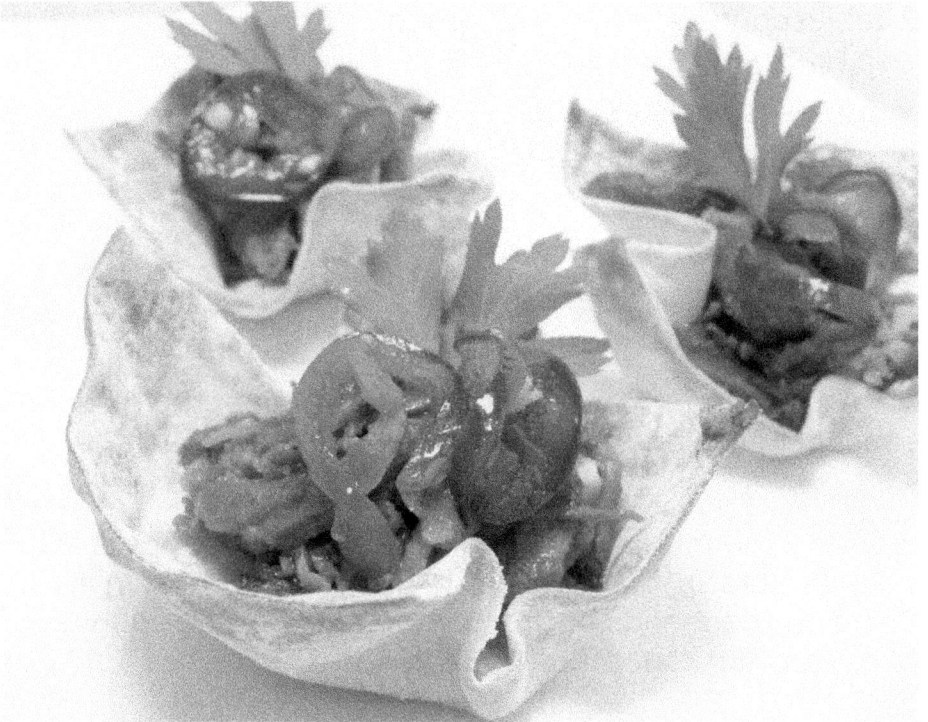

Southwestern Caprese Bites

Cooking Time:

10 minutes

Serve:2

Ingredients:

½ pound cherry tomatoes

1 tablespoon extra-virgin olive oil

½ pound bocconcini, drained

2 tablespoon fresh basil leaves

½ teaspoon chili powder

½ teaspoon ground cumin

¼ teaspoon garlic powder

Sea salt and ground black pepper, to taste

Directions:

1.Brush the cherry tomatoes with olive oil and transfer them to the cooking basket. Bake the cherry tomatoes at 400 degrees F for 4 minutes.

2.Assemble the bites by using a toothpick and skewer cherry tomatoes, bocconcini and fresh basil leaves.

3.Season with chili powder, cumin, garlic powder, salt and black pepper. Arrange on a nice serving platter Serve and enjoy!

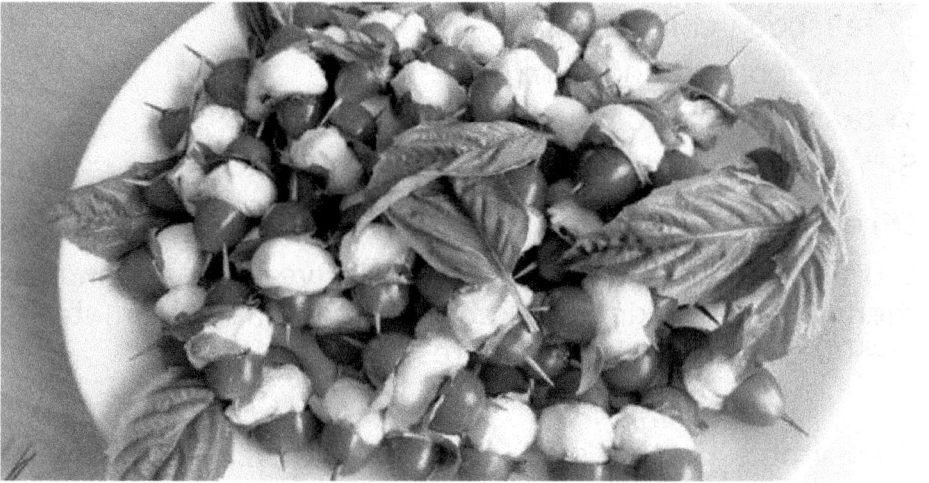

Salmon, Cheese and Cucumber Bites

Cooking Time:

15 minutes

Serve:3

Ingredients:

½ pound salmon

1 teaspoon extra-virgin olive oil

½ teaspoon onion powder

¼ teaspoon cumin powder

1 teaspoon granulated garlic

Sea salt and ground black pepper, to taste

2 ounces cream cheese

1 English cucumber, cut into 1- inch rounds

Directions:

1.Pat the salmon dry and drizzle it with olive oil. Season the salmon with onion powder, cumin, granulated garlic, salt and black pepper.

2.Transfer the salmon to the Air Fryer cooking basket. Cook the salmon at 400 degrees F for 5 minutes; turn the salmon over and continue to cook for 5 minutes more or until opaque.

3.Cut the salmon into bite- sized pieces. Spread 1 teaspoon of cream cheese on top of each cucumber slice; top each slice with a piece of salmon.

4.Insert a tiny party fork down the center to keep in place. Enjoy!

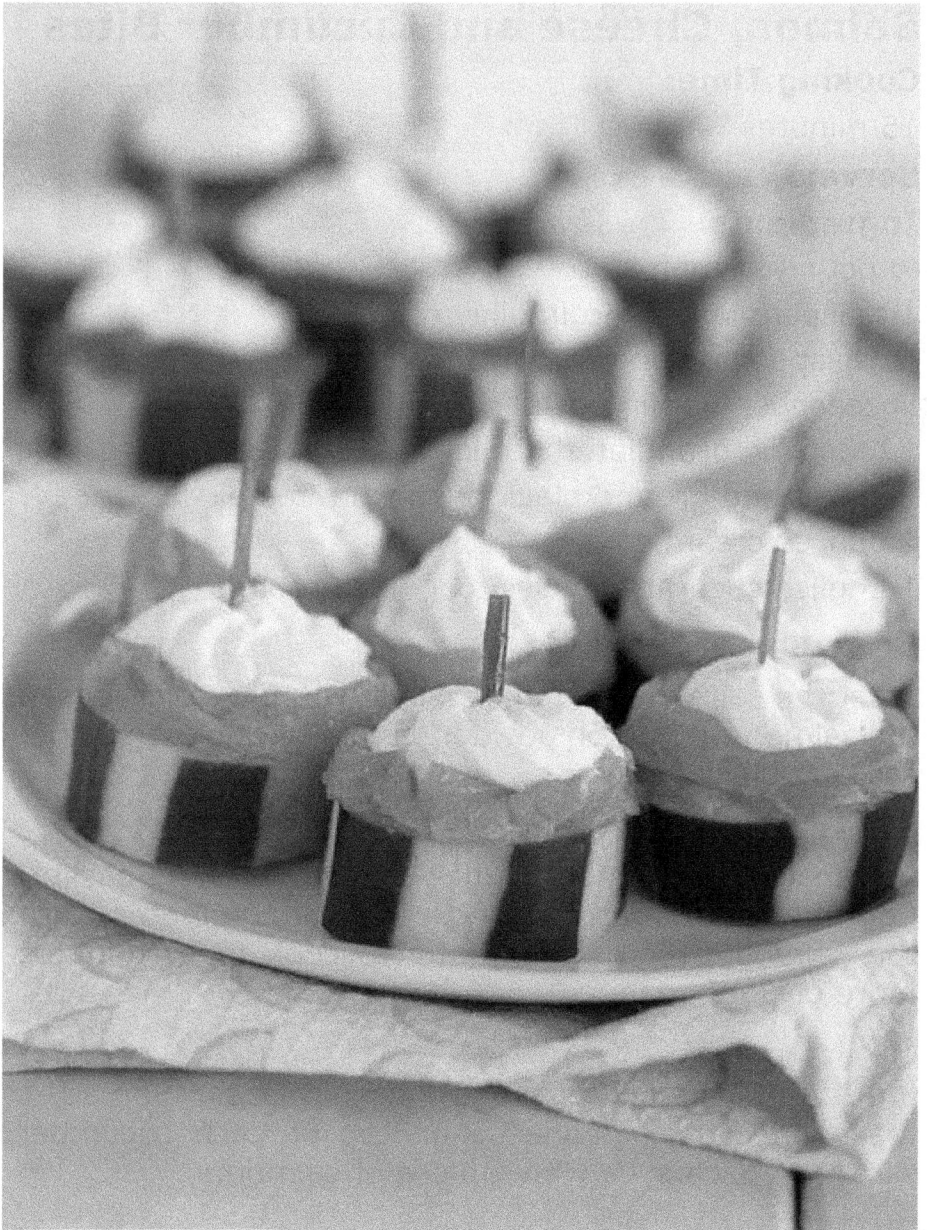

Mint Plantain Bites

Cooking Time:

10 minutes

Serve:3

Ingredients:

1pound plantains, peeled and cut into rounds

1 teaspoon coconut oil

A pinch of coarse sea salt

1 tablespoon mint leaves, chopped

Directions:

1.Start by preheating your Air Fryer to 350 degrees F. Brush the plantain rounds with coconut oil and sprinkle with coarse sea salt.

2.Cook the plantain rounds in the preheated Air Fryer for 5 minutes; shake the basket and cook for a further 5 minutes or until golden on the top.

3.Garnish with roughly chopped mint and serve. Enjoy!

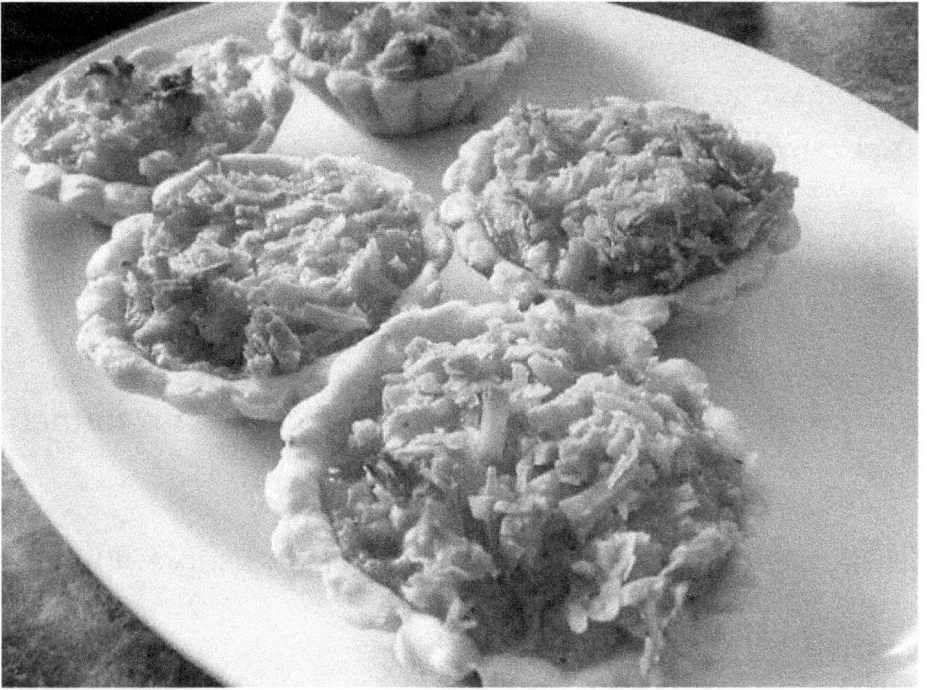

Paprika Potato Chips

Cooking Time:

50 minutes

Serve:3

Ingredients:

3 potatoes, thinly sliced

1 teaspoon sea salt

1 teaspoon garlic powder

1 teaspoon paprika

¼ cup ketchup

Directions

1.Add the sliced potatoes to a bowl with salted water. Let them soak for 30 minutes. Drain and rinse your potatoes.

2.Pat dry and toss with salt. Cook in the preheated Air Fryer at 400 degrees F for 15 minutes, shaking the basket occasionally.

3.Work in batches. Toss with the garlic powder and paprika. Serve with ketchup. Enjoy!

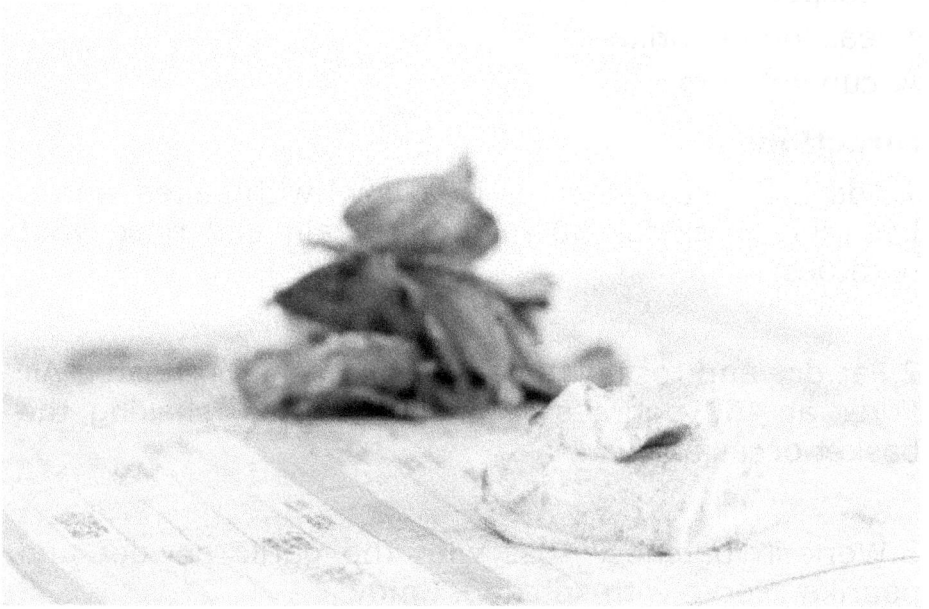

Sticky Glazed Wings

Cooking Time:

30 minutes

Serve:2

Ingredients:

½ pound chicken wings

1 tablespoon sesame oil

2 tablespoons brown sugar

1 tablespoon Worcestershire sauce

1 tablespoon hot sauce

1 tablespoon balsamic vinegar

Directions:

1.Brush the chicken wings with sesame oil and transfer them to the Air Fryer cooking basket.

2.Cook the chicken wings at 370 degrees F for 12 minutes; turn them over and cook for a further 10 minutes.

3.Meanwhile, bring the other ingredients to a boil in a saucepan; cook for 2 to 3 minutes or until thoroughly cooked.

4.Toss the warm chicken wings with the sauce and place them on a serving platter. Serve and enjoy!

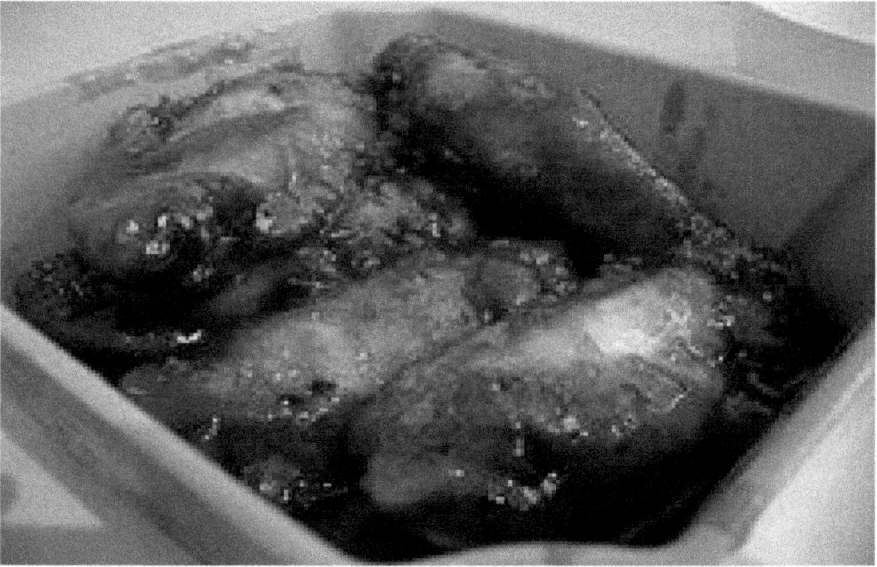

Asian Twist Chicken Wings

Cooking Time:
30 minutes
Serve:6
Ingredients:

1 ½ pounds chicken wings

2 teaspoons sesame oil Kosher salt and ground black pepper, to taste

2 tablespoons tamari sauce

1 tablespoon rice vinegar

2 garlic clove, minced

2 tablespoons honey

2 sun-dried tomatoes, minced

Directions:

1.Toss the chicken wings with the sesame oil, salt, and pepper.

2.Add chicken wings to a lightly greased baking pan. Roast the chicken wings in the preheated Air Fryer at 390 degrees F for 7 minutes.

3.Turn them over once or twice to ensure even cooking. In a mixing dish, thoroughly combine the tamari sauce, vinegar, garlic, honey, and sun-dried tomatoes.

4.Pour the sauce all over the chicken wings; bake an additional 5 minutes. Serve warm.

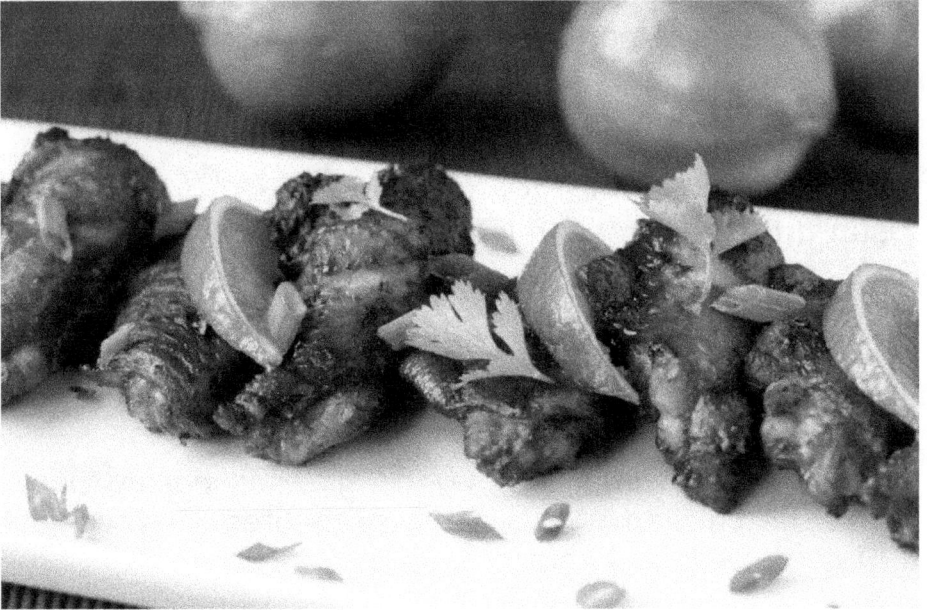

Beer-Battered Vidalia Onion Rings

Cooking Time:

15 minutes

Serve: 2

Ingredients:

½ cup all-purpose flour

½ teaspoon baking powder

¼ teaspoon cayenne pepper

¼ teaspoon dried oregano

Kosher salt and ground black pepper, to taste

1 large egg, beaten

¼ cup beer

1 cup crushed tortilla chips

½ pound Vidalia onions, cut into rings

Directions:

1. In a mixing bowl, thoroughly combine the flour, baking powder, cayenne pepper, oregano, salt, black pepper, egg and beer; mix to combine well.

2. In another shallow bowl, place the crushed tortilla chips. Dip the Vidalia rings in the beer mixture; then, coat the rings with the crushed tortilla chips, pressing to adhere.

3. Transfer the onion rings to the Air Fryer cooking basket and spritz them with a nonstick spray.

4. Cook the onion rings at 380 degrees F for about 8 minutes, shaking the basket halfway through the cooking time to ensure even browning. Serve and enjoy!

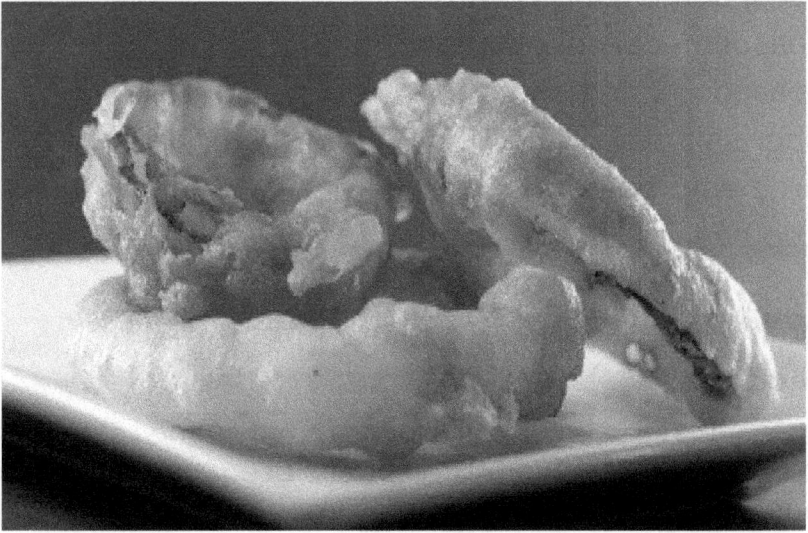

Coconut Banana Chips

Cooking Time:

10 minutes

Serve:2

Ingredients:

1 large banana, peeled and sliced
1 teaspoon coconut oil
¼ teaspoon ground cinnamon
A pinch of coarse salt
2 tablespoons coconut flakes

Directions:

1.Toss the banana slices with the coconut oil, cinnamon and salt.

2.Transfer banana slices to the Air Fryer cooking basket. Cook the banana slices at 375 degrees F for about 8 minutes, shaking the basket every 2 minutes.

3.Scatter coconut flakes over the banana slices and let banana chips cool slightly before serving. Enjoy!

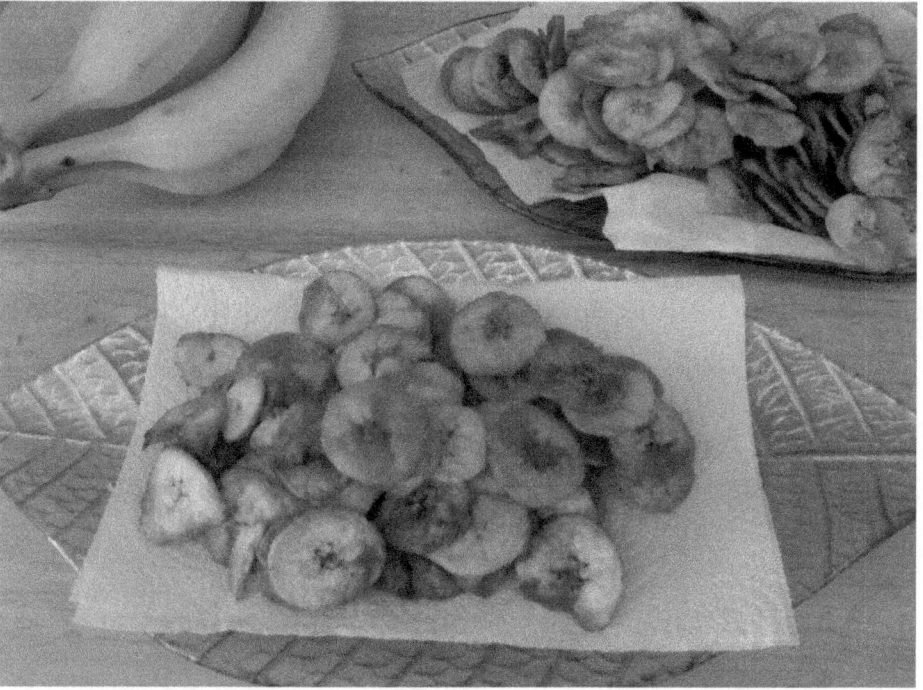

Eggplant Parm Chips

Cooking Time:

30 minutes

Serve:2

Ingredients:

½ pound eggplant, cut into rounds

Kosher salt and ground black pepper, to taste

½ teaspoon shallot powder

½ teaspoon porcini powder

½ teaspoon garlic powder

¼ teaspoon cayenne pepper

½ cup Parmesan cheese, grated

Directions:

1.Toss the eggplant rounds with the remaining ingredients until well coated on both sides.

2.Bake the eggplant chips at 400 degrees F for 15 minutes; shake the basket and continue to cook for 15 minutes more.

3.Let cool slightly, eggplant chips will crisp up as it cools. Enjoy!

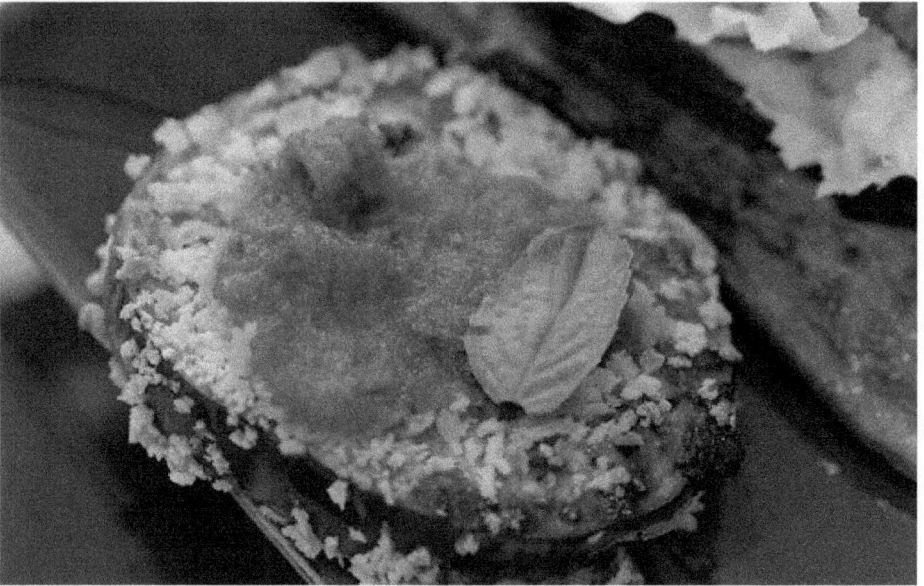

Mexican Crunchy Cheese Straws

Cooking Time:

15 minutes

Serve:4

Ingredients:

½ cup almond flour

¼ teaspoon xanthan gum

¼ teaspoon shallot powder

¼ teaspoon garlic powder

¼ teaspoon ground cumin

1 egg yolk, whisked

1 ounce Manchego cheese, grated

2 ounces Cotija cheese, grated

Directions:

Mix all ingredients until everything is well incorporated. Twist the batter into straw strips and place them on a baking mat inside your Air Fryer.

2.Cook the cheese straws in your Air Fryer at 360 degrees F for 5 minutes; turn them over and cook an additional 5 minutes.

3.Let the cheese straws cool before serving. Enjoy!

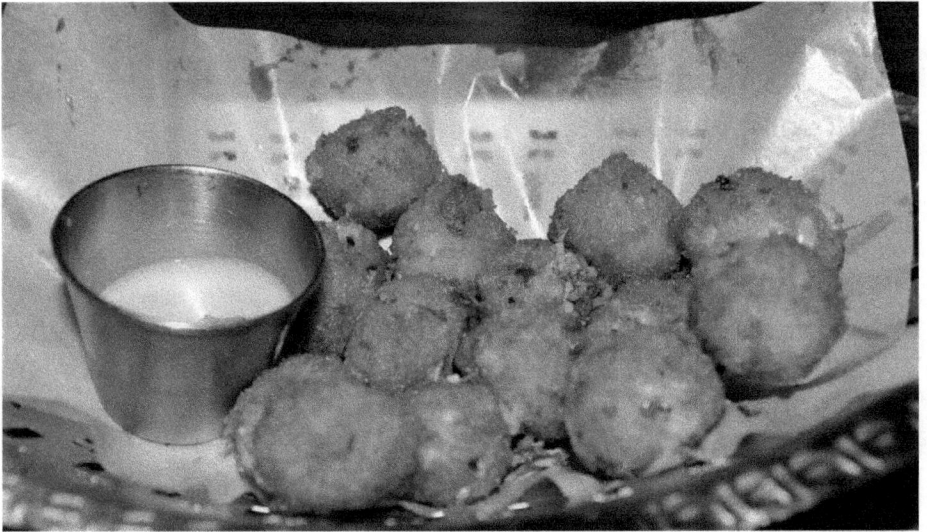

Greek-Style Deviled Eggs

Cooking Time:

20 minutes

Serve:4

Ingredients:
2 eggs
1 tablespoon chives, chopped
1 tablespoon parsley, chopped
2 tablespoons Kalamata olives, pitted and chopped
1 tablespoon Greek-style yogurt
1 teaspoon habanero pepper, seeded and chopped
Sea salt and crushed red pepper flakes, to taste

Directions:

Place the wire rack in the Air Fryer basket and lower the eggs onto the rack.

2.Cook the eggs at 260 degrees F for 15 minutes. Transfer the eggs to an ice-cold water bath to stop cooking. Peel the eggs under cold running water; slice them into halves, separating the whites and yolks.

3.Mash the egg yolks with the remaining ingredients and mix to combine. Spoon the yolk mixture into the egg whites and serve well chilled. Enjoy!

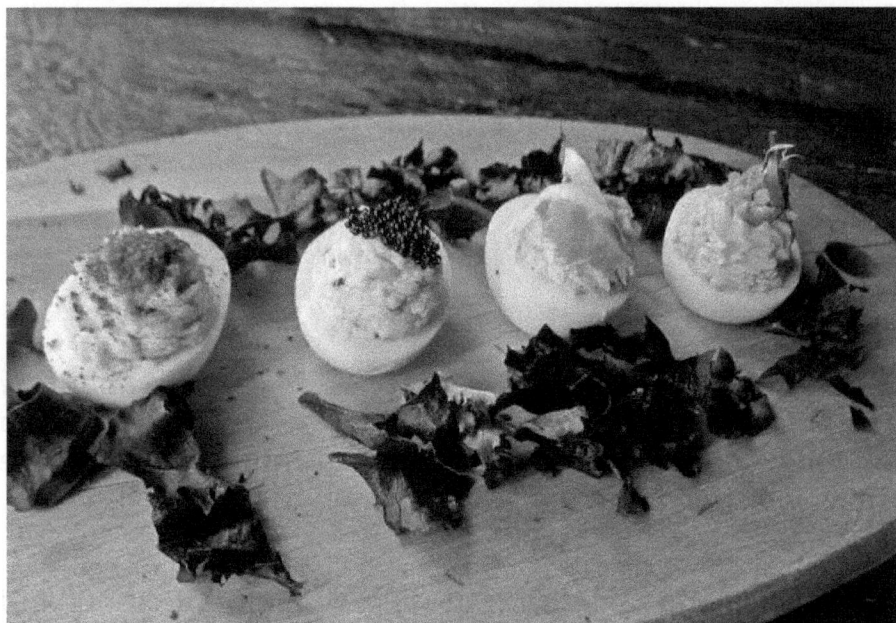

Puerto Rican Tostones

Cooking Time:

15 minutes

Serve:3

Ingredients:

1 ripe plantain, sliced

1 tablespoon sunflower oil

A pinch of grated nutmeg

A pinch of kosher salt

Directions:

1.Toss the plantains with the oil, nutmeg, and salt in a bowl.

2.Cook in the preheated Air Fryer at 400 degrees F for 10 minutes, shaking the cooking basket halfway through the cooking time.

3.Adjust the seasonings to taste and serve immediately.

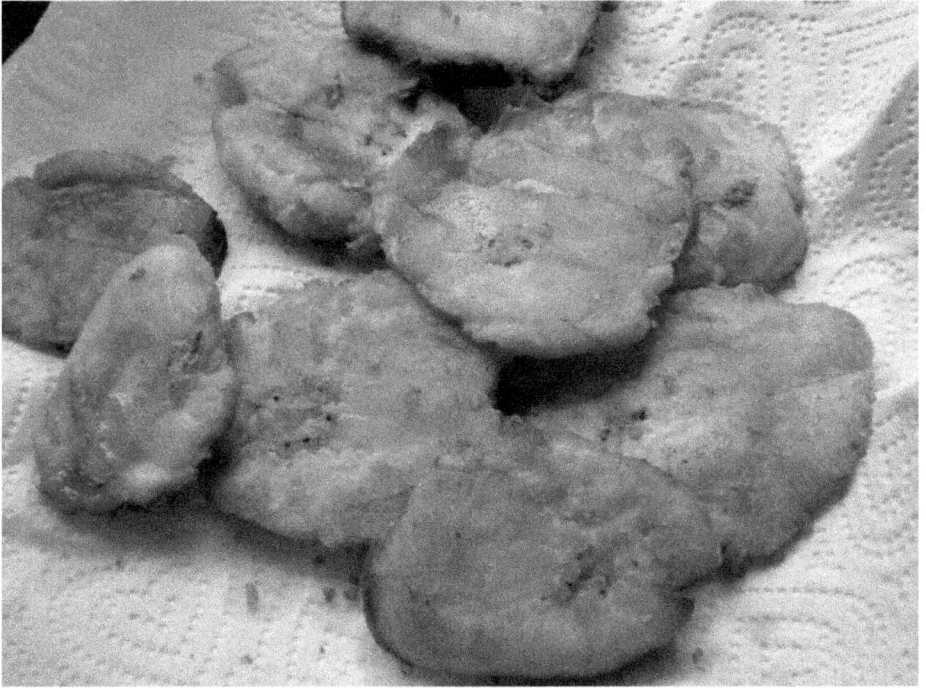

Green Bean Crisps

Cooking Time:

20 minutes

Serve:3

Ingredients:

1egg, beaten

¼ cup cornmeal

¼ cup parmesan, grated

1 teaspoon sea salt

½ teaspoon red pepper flakes, crushed

1 pound green beans

2 tablespoons grapeseed oil

Directions:

1.Ina mixing bowl, combine together the egg, cornmeal, parmesan, salt, and red pepper flakes; mix to combine well.

2.Dip the green beans into the batter and transfer them to the cooking basket. Brush with the grapeseed oil. Cook in the preheated Air Fryer at 390 degrees F for 4 minutes.

3.Shake the basket and cook for a further 3 minutes. Work in batches. Taste, adjust the seasonings and serve. Serve warm.

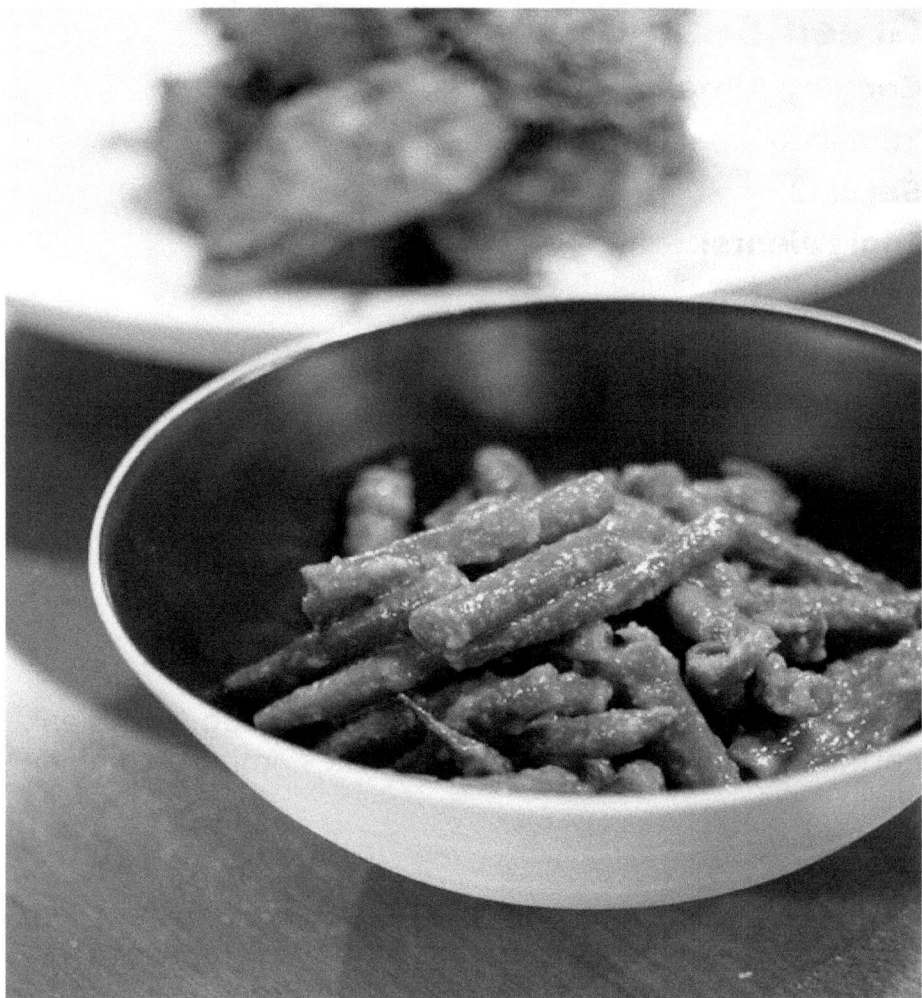

Quick and Easy Popcorn

Cooking Time:
20 minutes
Serve:4
Ingredients:

1tablespoons dried corn kernels

1 teaspoon safflower oil

Kosher salt, to taste

1 teaspoon red pepper flakes, crushed

Directions:

1.Add the dried corn kernels to the Air Fryer basket; brush with safflower oil.

2.Cook at 395 degrees F for 15 minutes, shaking the basket every 5 minutes. Sprinkle with salt and red pepper flakes. Enjoy!

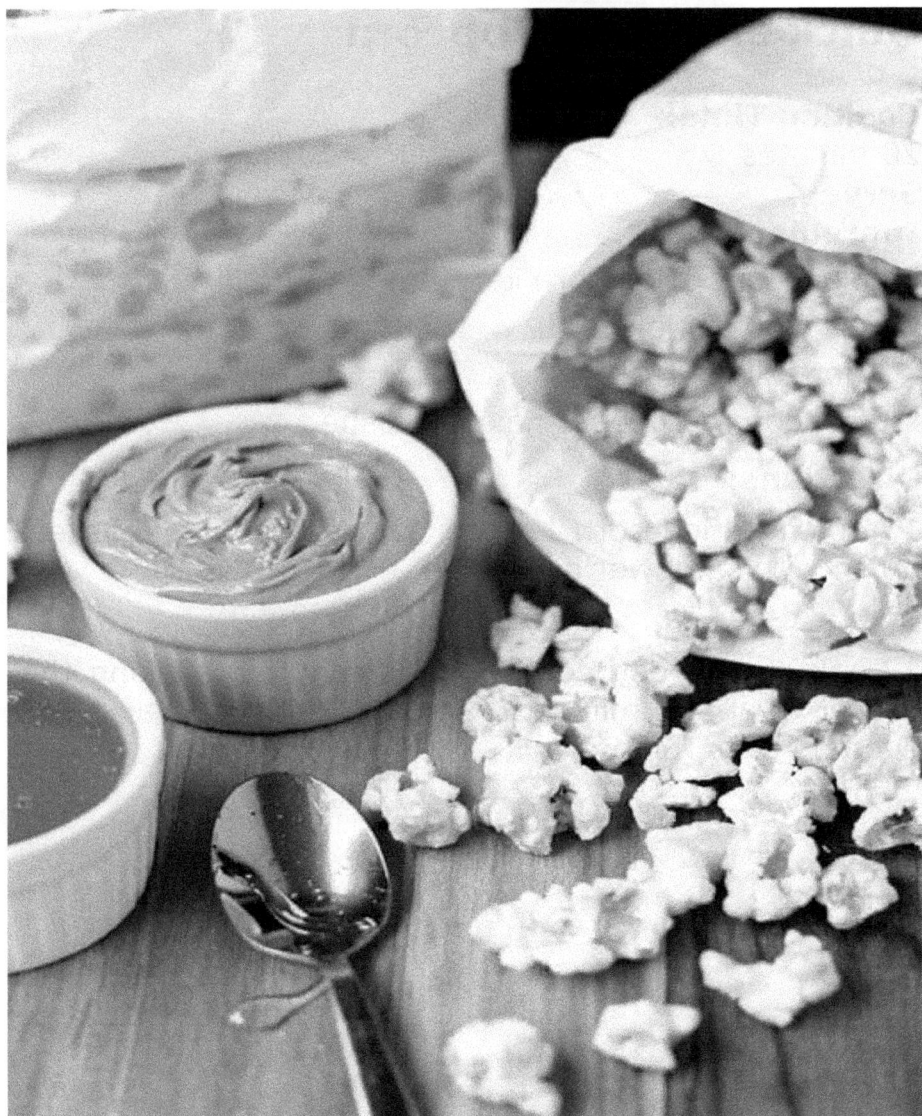

Homemade Ranch Tater Tots

Cooking Time:

15 minutes

Serve: 2

Ingredients:

½ pound potatoes, peeled and shredded

½ teaspoon hot paprika

½ teaspoon dried marjoram

1 teaspoon Ranch seasoning mix

2 tablespoons Colby cheese, finely grated about ⅓ cup

1 teaspoon butter, melted

Sea salt and ground black pepper, to taste

Directions:

1.In a mixing bowl, thoroughly combine all ingredients until everything is well incorporated.

2.Transfer your tater tots to a lightly greased Air Fryer cooking basket.

3.Cook your tater tots in the preheated Air Fryer at 400 degrees F for 12 minutes, shaking the basket halfway through the cooking time to ensure even browning. Serve and enjoy

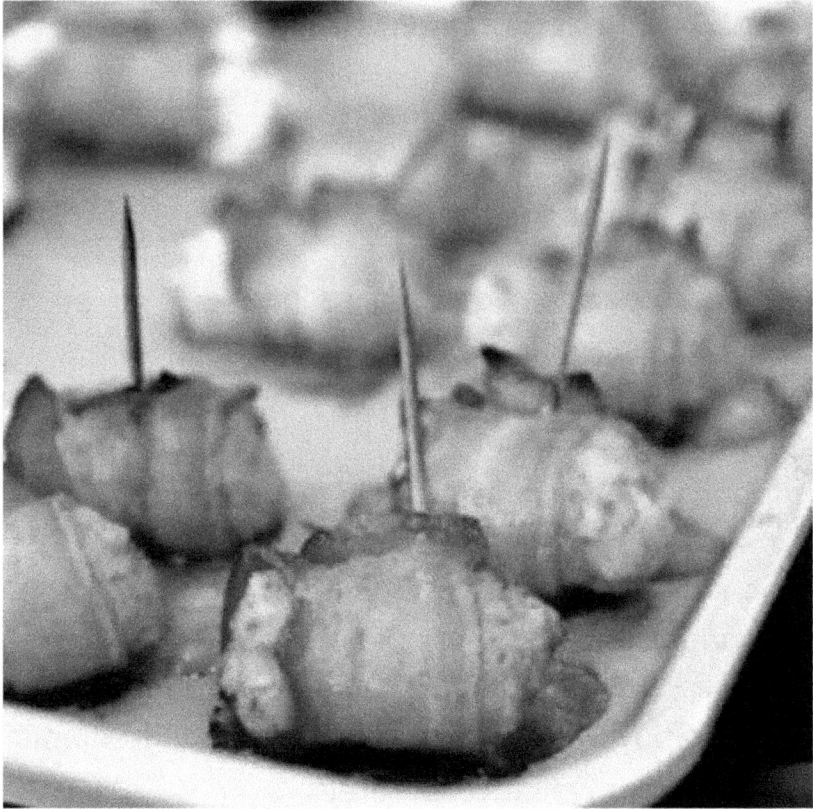

Barbecue Little Smokies

Cooking Time:

20 minutes

Serve:2

Ingredients:

1 pound beef cocktail wieners

10 ounces barbecue sauce

Directions:

1.Start by preheating your Air Fryer to 380 degrees F. Prick holes into your sausages using a fork and transfer them to the baking pan.

2.Cook for 13 minutes. Spoon the barbecue sauce into the pan and cook an additional 2 minutes. Serve with toothpicks. Enjoy!

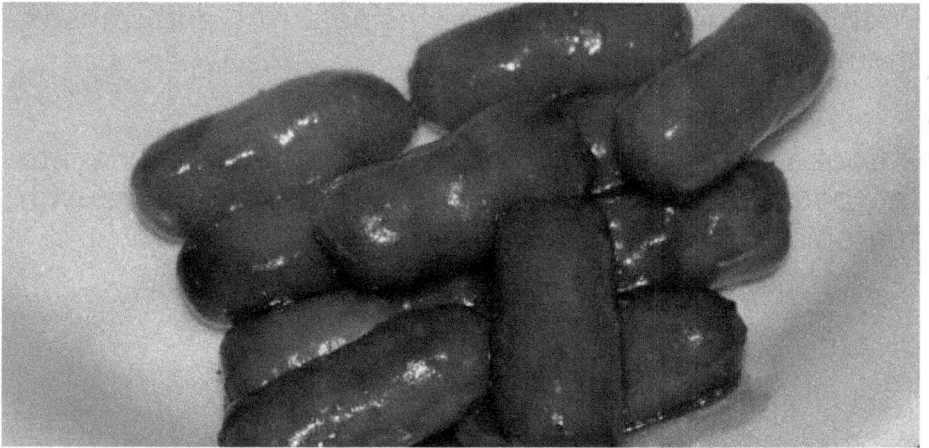

Baby Carrots with Asian Flair

Cooking time:

20 minutes

Serve:2

Ingredients:

1pound baby carrots

2 tablespoons sesame oil

½ teaspoon Szechuan pepper

1 teaspoon Wuxiang powder Five-spice powder

1 tablespoon honey

1 large garlic clove, crushed

1 1-inch piece fresh ginger root, peeled and grated

2 tablespoons tamari sauce

Directions:

1.Start by preheating your Air Fryer to 380 degrees F. Toss all ingredients together and place them in the Air Fryer basket.

2.Cook for 15 minutes, shaking the basket halfway through the cooking time. Enjoy!

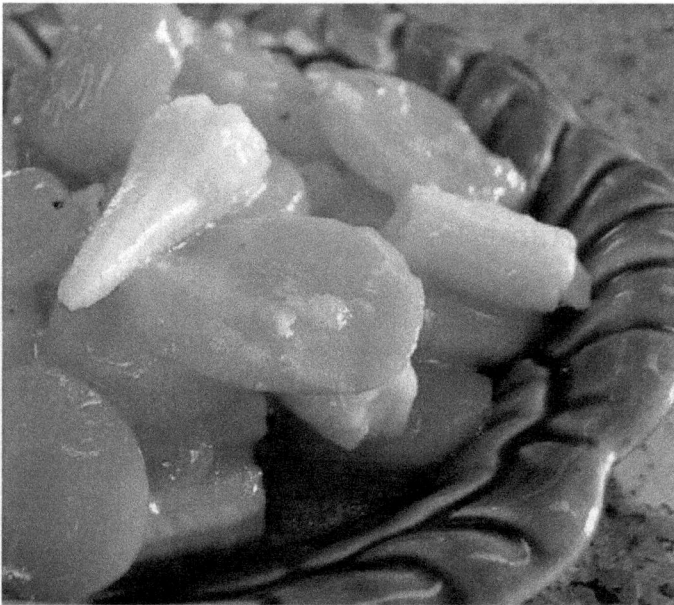

Greek-Style Squash Chips

Cooking Time:

25 minutes

Serve:4

Ingredients:
½ cup seasoned breadcrumbs
½ cup Parmesan cheese, grated
Sea salt and ground black pepper, to taste
¼ teaspoon oregano
2 yellow squash, cut into slices
2 tablespoons grapeseed oil

Sauce:

½ cup Greek-style yogurt

1 tablespoon fresh cilantro, chopped

1 garlic clove, minced Freshly ground black pepper, to your liking

Directions:
1.In a shallow bowl, thoroughly combine the seasoned breadcrumbs, Parmesan, salt, black pepper, and oregano.

2.Dip the yellow squash slices in the prepared batter, pressing to adhere.

3.Brush with the grapeseed oil and cook in the preheated Air Fryer at 400 degrees F for 12 minutes. Shake the Air Fryer basket periodically to ensure even cooking. Work in batches.

4.While the chips are baking, whisk the sauce ingredients; place in your refrigerator until ready to serve. Enjoy!

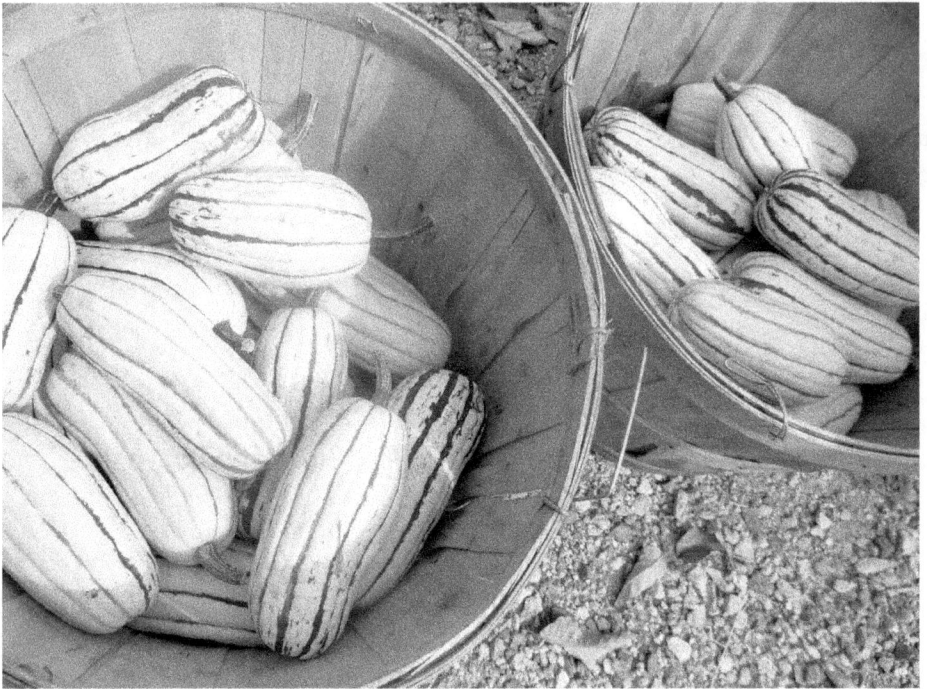

Cajun Cheese Sticks

Cooking Time:

15 minutes

Serve:4

Ingredients:

½ cup all-purpose flour

2 eggs

½ cup parmesan cheese, grated

1 tablespoon Cajun seasonings

8 cheese sticks, kid- friendly ¼ cup ketchup

Directions:

1.To begin, set up your breading station. Place the all-purpose flour in a shallow dish. In a separate dish, whisk the eggs.

2.Finally, mix the parmesan cheese and Cajun seasoning in a third dish.

3.Start by dredging the cheese sticks in the flour; then, dip them into the egg. Press the cheese sticks into the parmesan mixture, coating evenly.

4.Place the breaded cheese sticks in the lightly greased Air Fryer basket. Cook at 380 degrees F for 6 minutes. Serve with ketchup and enjoy!

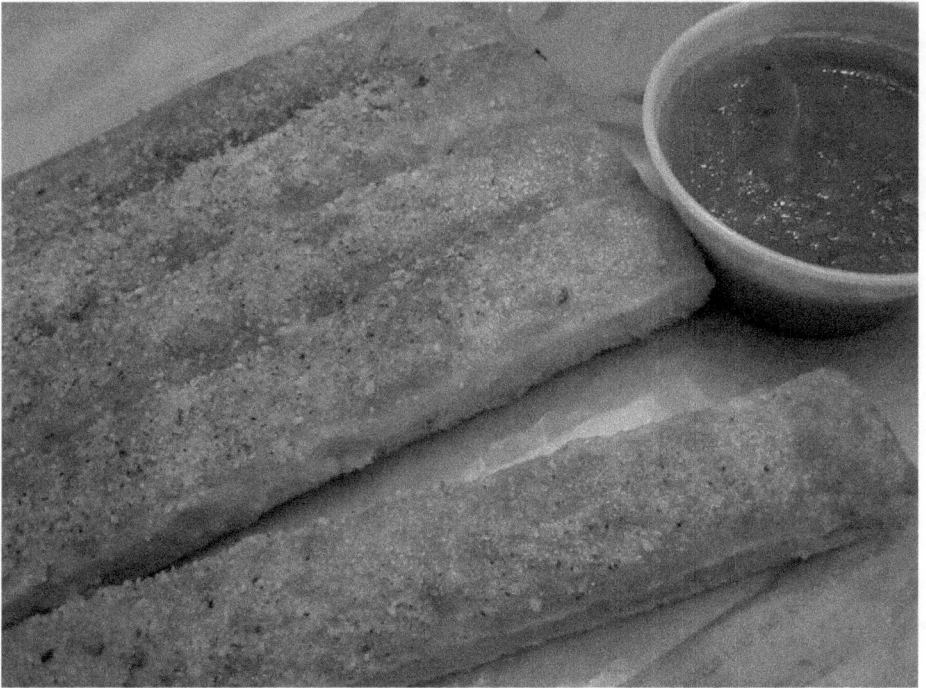

Kale Chips with White Horseradish Mayo

Cooking Time:

10 minutes

Serve:4

Ingredients:

1 cups loosely packed kale

1 teaspoon sesame oil

Sea salt and ground black pepper, to taste

1 teaspoon sesame seeds, lightly toasted

1 ounce mayonnaise

1 teaspoon prepared white horseradish

Directions:

1.Toss the kale pieces with sesame oil, salt and black pepper.

2.Cook the kale pieces at 370 degrees F for 2 minutes; shake the basket and continue to cook for 2 minutes more.

3.Meanwhile, make the horseradish mayo by whisking the mayonnaise and prepared horseradish. Let cool slightly, kale chips will crisp up as it cools. Sprinkle toasted sesame seeds over the kale chips.

4.Serve the kale chips with the horseradish mayo. Enjoy!

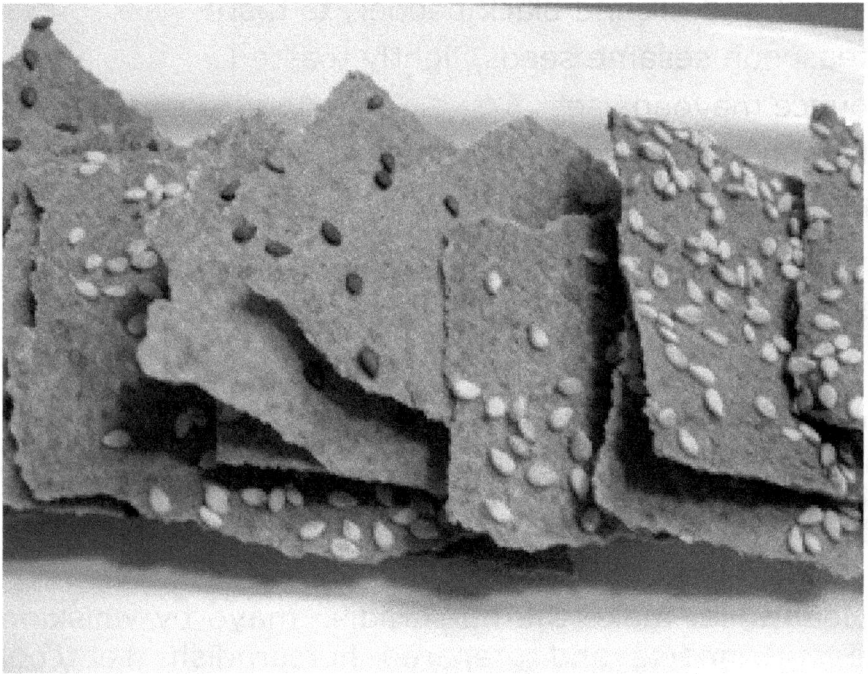

Mexican Cheesy Zucchini Bites

Cooking Time:

25 minutes

Serve: 4

Ingredients:

1large-sized zucchini, thinly sliced
½ cup flour
¼ cup yellow cornmeal
1 egg, whisked
½ cup tortilla chips, crushed
½ cup Queso Añejo, grated
Salt and cracked pepper, to taste

Directions:

1.Pat dry the zucchini slices with a kitchen towel. Mix the remaining ingredients in a shallow bowl; mix until everything is well combined.

2.Dip each zucchini slice in the prepared batter. Cook in the preheated Air Fryer at 400 degrees F for 12 minutes, shaking the basket halfway through the cooking time.

3.Work in batches until the zucchini slices are crispy and golden brown. Enjoy!

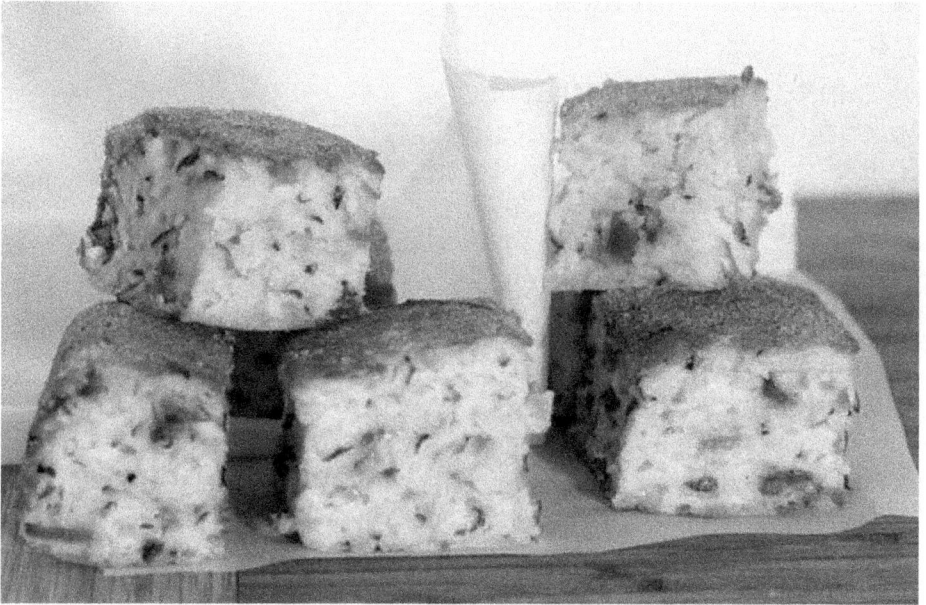

www.ingramcontent.com/pod-product-compliance
Lightning Source LLC
Chambersburg PA
CBHW050757030426
42336CB00012B/1858